Life Stories
Observation of a Physician

Life Stories
Observation of a Physician

Dr. Nowsheen Sharmin Purabi

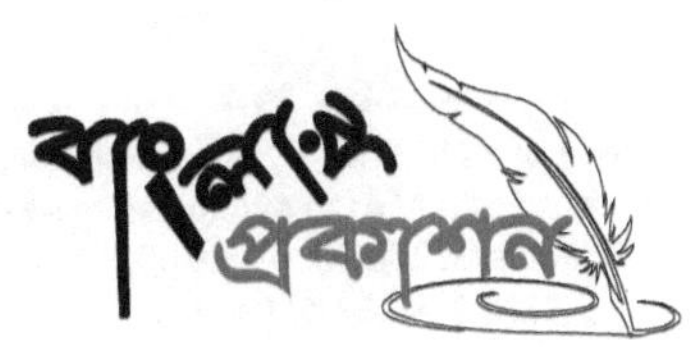

Life Stories
Observation of a Physician

Dr. Nowsheen Sharmin Purabi

First Published
January 2018

Publisher
Ahsan Al Azad
Banglar Prokashon

Office
106 Fakirapool (2nd Floor), Motijheel, Dhaka-1000, Bangladesh
Cell: 01977 753 753
Email: info@banglarkobita.com
Wabesite: www.BanglarKobita.com

Copyright:
Dr. Nowsheen Sharmin Purabi

Cover Deisgn:
Mohammad Toufiq Hossain Khan

Compose:
A Cube Business Service

Print:
Nitol Print

Price
Tk. 200.00

Life Stories: Observation of a Physician by Dr. Nowsheen Sharmin Purabi
Published by Ahasan Al Azad of Banglar Prokashon
Price Tk. 200.00, US $ 6.00
ISBN: 978-984-92698-5-4

Preface

As Doctor Nowsheen Sharmin Purabi is a socially concious physician and possessing woman entity in heart and mind, so she thinks of essentiality of writing the book 'Life Stories'. Not only the health service but also the attempt to make the women health conscious is her professional responsibility. The composition of 'Life Stories' is the outburst of such contemplation.

These writings are not simply stories. She tried here to represent the facts before the readers like telling the true stories. She analyses here the complex issues of medical field in linear descriptions along with the possible remedies of problems. The style of telling stories reflects her scholastic efficiency. I think, as the writer is a woman so she could easily enter inside the mind of a woman like the wave of river water. Her language and sentences are very consistent and adept in continuity of the facts. She produces the tough situations simply through these stories.

I believe this book will be a milestone addition for creating social conciousness. All of us should have one copy of this book in collection. My advice to all the guardians to read every story of the book attentively. There are 32 stories in the book.The writer explicitly presents 32 health problems here.

We have to face such circumstances due to traditional views, illiteracy and neglegence. To change the time we have to lead our life to the light leaving the darkness behind. Men and women should be prompted by sense of conciousness and responsibility. Then it will be possible to have a healthy baby and safe mother as the gift.

The writer has given a clear guideline to our views as described in the story no. 33 of Life Stories. In the concluding stage of the book 'Let's Change Ourselves' reflects her sufficient efficiency.We find out her firm and bright determination and willingness in loud voice. I hope overall success and wide circulation of her book.

Nasrin Nayem
Poet and Story writer, Former Head Mistress
Viqarun Nisa Noon School and College

Acknowledgement

Each story of "Life Stories" is a fact. For the sake of privacy, the names of the patients are not disclosed here. I am grateful to my teachers, collegues and well wishers. I have got the scope to write the "Life Stories" having the opportunity to work with them.

I believe it is not only the poverty but also the lack of awareness; family and social support are the causes for female reproductive health care problems of Bangladesh. Most of the women are shy, hesitant, and ignorant and in some cases financially dependent and unable to make self-decision.

I dream of such a world where repetition of such incident will be decreased. Health awareness will be expanded in personal, family and social level. At the same time people will expand the hands for cooperation and sympathy. The world then will be a safe home for our future generation.

Dhaka   Dr. Nowsheen Sharmin Purabi
Date: 01.01.2018

A letter to my daughter…

Dear Purnata

Your inauguration to the light of the world has given me a new dynamism in my work field, extended my respoliabilities as a physician. The exclamation of all the children in the world seems to be your weeping to me. Observing the sick, helpless and under previledged female patients, I pray to God not to face such a tough situation by you.

Some stanza of the poem of the poet Sukanta is recited in my mind,

'I'll remove all the trashes trying heart and soul till breathing last;

I'll make the world suitable to live for the children.

It's my strong commitment to the new born.'

There is a proverb 'What mind does not know, eyes cannot see'. It's my little effort to make you aware, self confident, fighting soldier.

As I am nourishing you with utmost care and sincerety I hope that you'll address more responsibility to your next generation than that of me.

Live sound and safe.
I dedicate "Life Stories" to you.

Your mother

1. Life Stories

Sonia, the mother of two children, was 22 years old.

Her first issue was a daughter of five years.

The daughter was born in her home. A sound and nice baby she is. The son was born after five years in her home also. The baby delayed to cry after the birth. So they visited the doctor and hospitalized.The child appeared to be normal after a vast medical treatment and spending huge amount of money for that time.

Six months had passed but the child could not hold the neck straight but cries only. The baby was then one year old and he could not make any sound or sit. The mother took care of the baby all the day. Instead of repeated visit to doctors there was no progress. As the mother took care of the baby all the day there was no scope to take care of her. She had become shattered both physically and mentally. But why did it happen?

If breathing is difficult for the new born baby during the time of delivery or pregnancy period then the brain of the child becomes injured due to insufficiency of oxygen. That's why, during the time of delivery, a new born can not cry. In medical term, it is defined as 'Cerebral Palsy'.

Sonia had to go forward admitting this problem with cooperation of family and society. Rehabilitation centers had been established for the physical and mental development of such children. But it was not sufficient to meet the demand. The state and the society have a big role to help such children making the availability of health and medical facilities. Grant from the government can be arranged so that the families do not face any financial trouble in taking care of such children.

Such types of children never get cured completely. But their conditions can be improved by providing them with medical treatment and physio-therapy. In order to avoid such problems, the delivery of new born baby should be performed in a heath care centers instead of home.

2. Life Stories

Mother came to the physician taking eighteen years old Shoma with her. Her daughter was a college student.

The doctor asked the question, 'What's the problem?' The mother informed that the menstruation of her daughter had not yet been started. Her younger daughter was then fifteen and her menstruation had started since at age of eleven.

No physical and mental problem was diagnosed. As the girl was unmarried, ultrasonogram was done instead of any internal examination. The report was similar to prediction. 'Mullerian Agenesis'which refers to non-formation of uterus in the body of the girl. It caused nonestablishment of her menstruation.

If uterus is absent then it is not possible to grow it newly. The mother and the girl had to comply with this reality. This is similar to that problem where some people born without a leg or legs and without a hand or hands. It is not possible to grow or transplant the uterus from other donor.

As the girl was on study, she needed to continue it. In case of marriage of the girl the probable bridegroom to be informed of the disability frankly as child bearing would never be possible for her but would be able to maintain physical relation with the male partner.

Sometimes the orifice of the vagina remains closed which may be opened in surgical intervention.

The girl should be given proper mental support
by all.

Key Message:
If menstruation of any child does not start within the age of 16 years, the child is required to visit the doctor.

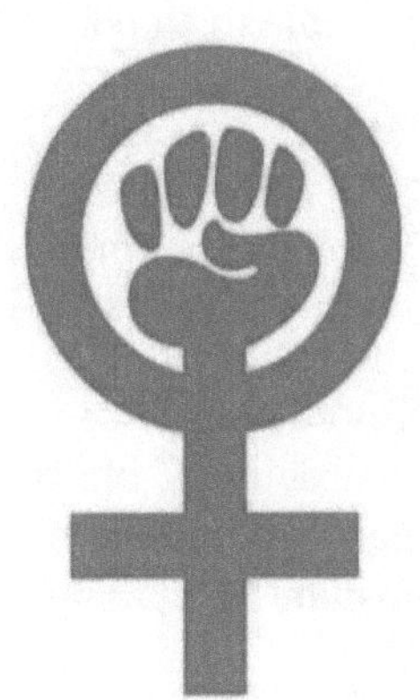

3. Life Stories

It was early morning.
Jesmin, about 26 years old pregnant lady was suffering from severe labour pain. Observing her physical condition she was taken to nearby small clinic by her family members.

After physical examination, the doctor told that the condition of the patient was serious. They arranged emergency delivery of the new born by C-section. A healthy baby was delivered. The joy of all the family members knew no bound.

Just after sometime, they could know that the life of the pleasure giver mother of the child was at stake. The post delivery bleeding of the mother was going on increasingly. Under such a circumstance, the doctor sewed the uterus (Mattress Suture) and tied the artery of uterus (Uterine Artery). But the bleeding was not stopped. Then the doctor removed partial uterus (Sub Total Hysterectomy) through surgery. Bleeding could not be stopped after applying all the possible procedures. The patient was lying down to death gradually. Finding no other alternative the patient was shifted to medical college hospital (Tertiary Care Center).

The family members of the patient had become nearly mad. The doctor assured them as he could and adviced to pray to Allah. A big artery of the patient (Internal Iliac Artery) was tied through the operative procedure. At last it was possible to stop bleeding.

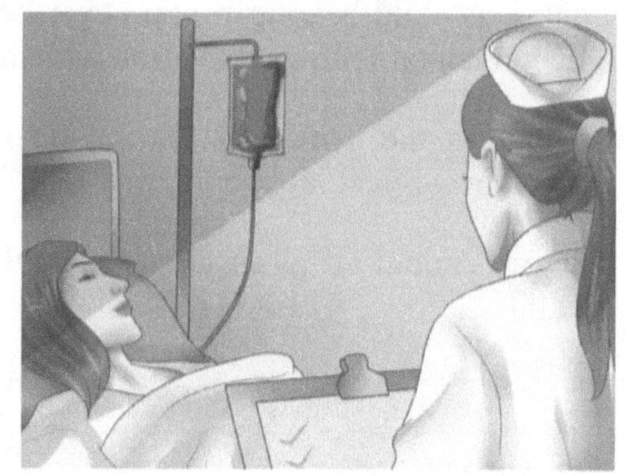

Jesmin was kept in observation in the hospital for 7 days. She then started to lead a normal life.

Key Message:
Post delivery bleeding is one of the main reasons for high rate of maternal death which may be possible to reduce taking the mother to hospital and taking medical care rapidly.

4. Life Stories

Shirin Akter, 23 years old, had also dream like some other ladies to form a happy family with husband and children.

She tried to be pregnant since one year after their marriage. But they could not conceive even after 5 years of their marriage. At last, she visited a doctor with the hope of a child. Her dream was to be a mother after receiving the treatment.

Doctor performed different investigations. Ultrasonography showed that, there was a cyst in her left ovary. The doctor removed the cyst by laparoscopic surgery. The sample was sent for histopathological test. Report shows "Mucinous Cyst Adenoma". As it was a benign tumor so the doctor assured the patient and the patient returned home after recovery.

The patient Shirin Akter had to come again to the doctor. Then the problems were breathing difficulty, swelling of abdomen and problem in walking. Laparoscopic surgery was performed for the second time. Ovarian cyst was found in same side which was bigger than the previous one. This time huge amount of mucinous fluid was draind during surgery. Again the sample was sent for histopathological investigation. It repeated the same as before and the patient also returned home after recovery.

No sooner had it passed 3 months then the patient had to face the same problem and visited doctor with same complain. At this stage the doctor consulted with an Oncologist. But the Oncologist discouraged for chemotherapy as it was a benign tumor.

The condition of the patient began to deteriorate. The doctor again decided to undergo a surgical procedure (laparotomy) and it was found that the opposite ovary was also involved. Then the affected part of the ovary was removed keeping the non-affected portion and the sample was sent for histopathological test which delivered the report "Mucinous Cyst Adenocarcinoma". Then the oncologist prescribed chemotherapy.

After applying the 6 cycles of chemotherapy the patient was reinvestigated and found no residual cyst. But there were some liquid substances deposited inside the abdomen. The patient was all but sound. But her menstruation process remained suspended.

When the patient was leading almost sound life getting rid of cancer, at that time the expectation to have a child was developed in her mind once again. When the doctor tried to convince her, she argued that, as her uterus was kept intact, she may proceed for a child bearing. But her ovary could not be saved which is essential for production of oocyte and it is an important element in child bearing process.

Although she could get rid of her survival exigency, the dream of Shirin Akter to become a mother remained as a dream only. It was one of the precious dreams of her life.

Key Message:
Cancer may be cured if it is diagnosed at a primary stage.

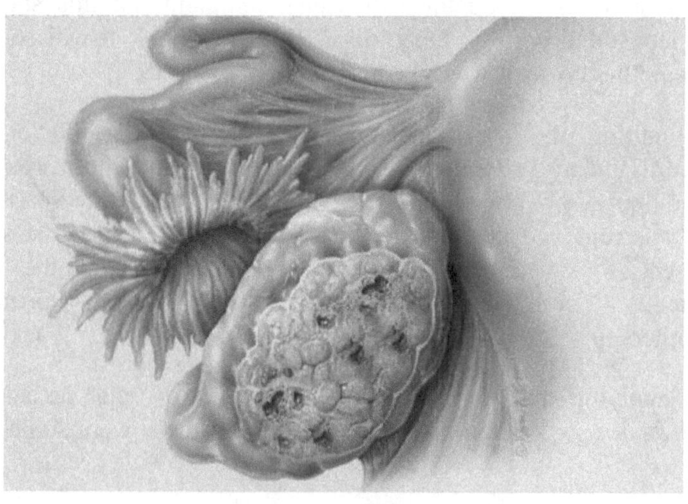

5. Life Stories

Trisna a girl of 20 years old was admitted to the hospital with severe pain in her abdomen being physically abused by her husband while she was pregnant for six months.

Three years ago she left her father's family and got married to her husband. She was a garments worker and her husband a day labor. She had the responsibility of running the family by her job, taking care of husband, father-in-law and mother-in-law in the family. When the poor father could not pay the dowry money completely then she had to be a victim of physical and mental tortures.

One year ago under the pressure created by the husband and mother-in-law she had to experience an induced abortion of her pregnancy. For the sake of being a mother, she had to bear all the pressures silently which were created by the husband, mother-in-law, the family and also from the job. In the six months of her pregnancy, she was tortured by her husband. As a consequence, she had to loss her child forever and had to remove her uterus due to severe damage in order to save her life.

The bleeding from uterus was profuse and if the uterus would not be removed, Trisna might have died. The torture of husband ended her dream of becoming a mother forever. She would be childless forever.

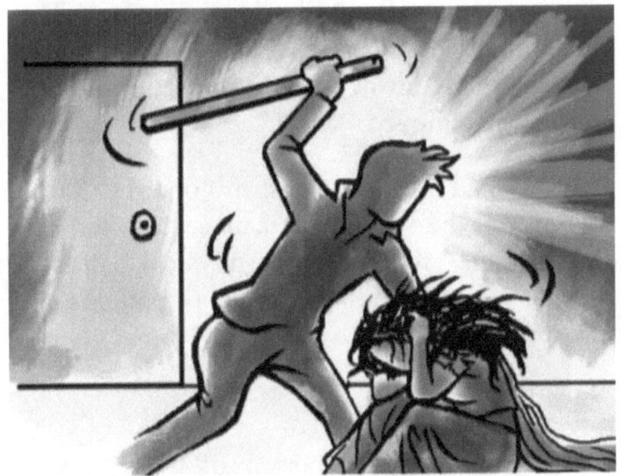

Key Message:
Let all types of violence against the women be stopped.

6. Life Stories

Saleha, a young lady of 21 years old came from a lower middle class family, had been married for 3 years. She had a daughter of 2 years old.

She visited a doctor with a complaint of irregular menstruation for seven months.

An elder sister and a brother brought her with them to the doctor. It seemed that they love their sister very much. When she was asked about her husband, she informed that he was bad and engaged in various evil activities like stealing, hijacking etc. He was in prison at the time.

Their financial condition was very bad. Brothers and sisters were maintaining her family. She used to work in garments earlier. She was unable to work because of illness for the last 6 months. The financial condition of her brother and sister was at a stake for undergoing medical treatment at various public and private hospitals along with expenses of medical investigations.

After being tested it was diagnosed that the girl had been suffering from a disease called "Chorio carcinoma." The girl was not cured after treatment twice at earlier. The doctor advised to remove her uterus. According to the decision of Saleha and her brother and sister her uterus was removed.

The lady had to give 6 bags of blood. For further medical treatment she was sent to the specialized cancer hospital. The girl came to the doctor several times to report her physical status. The love, respect, trust, confidence and blessings of many patients like her are the inspiration for us to walk on our way.

Key Message:
If a regular monthly period of a girl becomes irregular and other physical symptoms are noticed, then immediately she should have a doctor's consultation.

7. Life Stories

Mahima, 25 years old blind. She had become completely blind from a severe disease gradually through the last 15 years. She was literate.

She was married to another fellow young man of 28 years of age. He was also blind by birth.

What a strange matching! Both formed a family with happiness and sorrows. Their love was so deep that they thought that if they had a healthy child, it would be a partner of their sorrows in the future. Thinking of that she had become pregnant.

During her pregnancy, she came to the hospital for the first time at 9 months of pregnancy; her water bag surrounding the baby was ruptured 12 hours ago. The baby was in a risky situation inside the womb, so the baby was delivered by Caesarean section.

The new born died after two weeks of birth due to dyspnoea. Dreams of blind couples were broken down.

Mahima was really great. She wanted to take a big responsibility, the hope to give birth to a child inspite of her blind life who could be the means of their happiness and support in future.

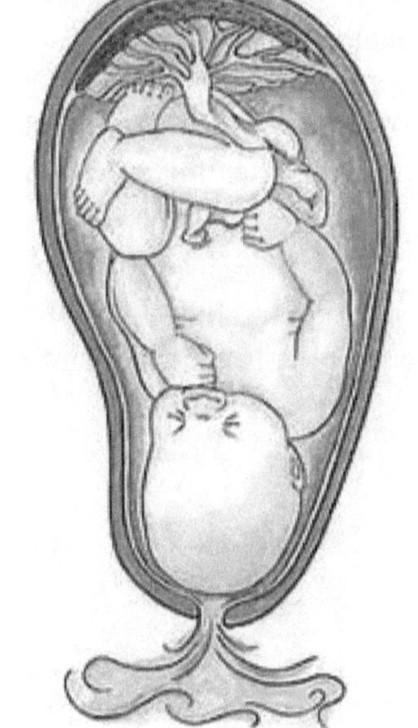

Thereafter, I do not know any more news of them; and do not know whether Mahima could have been a mother later?

Key Message:
Regular health checkup is neeeded during pregnancy for the delivery of a healthy baby.

8. Life Stories

Taslima, eighteen years old, came to the doctor's chamber during 37 weeks of her pregnancy.

She looked like a girl of an aristocratic family. It was found in investigation that the baby in the womb was very small. At the same time, the girl was suffering from pregnancy induced high blood pressure which was not controlled by medication. Urgent delivery of the baby was decided by Caesarean section. A lovely female baby was born.

Three days later, the girl went to her home with discharge certificate. While she was in the hospital, a gentle man was found lying on her bed. Besides, no other relatives could be seen. That guy was introduced as the cousin of the girl.

Actually, the girl had no relation with the guy. The girl was unmarried.

The girl who had become a mother in such a way, was supposed to be busy in class and studies in a university just after crossing her college level. As a risk of being a mother at a younger age, it could lead her to death.

And who was the baby that was born? Was it possible for the child to grow in a healthy environment with all necessary supports?

Key Message:
To prevent adolescent pregnancy, it is needed to give adequate health education to the child and nurture family values and understanding.

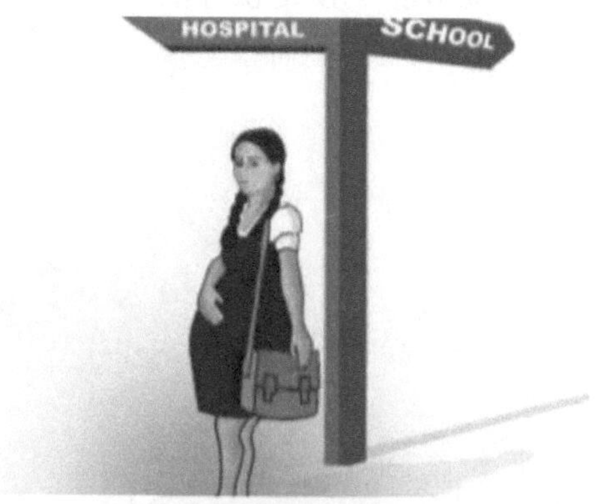

9. Life Stories

A simple, poor farmer father came to the doctor with his 16/17 years old daughter who lost her mother. Her name was Halima.
The father reported in crying voice that his daughter's family was being broken. The people of her father-in-law's house were thinking her a transgender as she had no menstruation yet then at all.

While doctor talked to Halima, she said in a loud voice that she's all right. She is not a hermaphrodite. The doctor examined her and found that her female organs were present but it was just like the kids. Then she was investigated with ultrasonogram and Karyo typing and it was diagnosed that she was a patient of Turner's syndrome (Turner's syndrome, Karyo typing 45X0).

The girl would never have menstruation and she would not be a mother. Her family life was endangered. Today or tomorrow the marital relation would break down.

Provisional hormonal treatment had been given to prevent her divorce right then so that it started bleeding like menstruation. It happened as expected. Everyone was happy of her father-in-law's house. Halima was rescued from the danger of this expedition. But it was a temporary treatment, not long-term.

Doctor explained the genetic problems to her. She must comply with her congenital problem. She would not be dependent on her father in law's house; even the poor father also would not be able to help her in any way. She should be self-dependent. Halima was not literate.

The doctor encouraged her to learn sewing to be self-sufficient. But she did not have money to be trained up. She was arranged to provide the training with financial assistance. In six months she learned good work. At first she used to work on other's machine. Later, she was initially financed for buying a sewing machine in installment. Slowly the rest of all was done by Halima. One day she informed that her husband had been married again, so she took care of her own work in full swing, not at home of co-wife. She was then the owner of 'Halima Tailors'. Not only that, she had established a nursery for her day-laborer farmer father. Then she was fully selfsufficient.

She often came to meet the doctor. In love for the doctor, she came with gift items like mango, vegetable of the field and flower plants.

There are many ill fated girls in our society who are living with troubles due to lack of proper guidance. We should provide proper guidance of rehabilitation along with treatment of these patients. Because people are for the people.

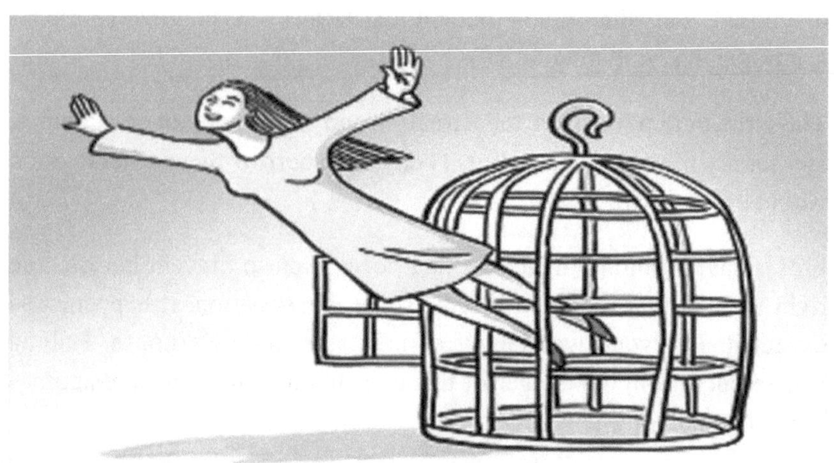

10. Life Stories

One day a patient came to the hospital in a critical condition.

She was pregnant, 8 days ago, her water bag was ruptured, the baby died in the womb. Operation was performed after arranging blood for transfusion.

During the surgery uterus was found gangrenous. The dead baby was delivered after cutting the green colored uterus. The bones of the baby had been entered inside the uterine wall.

Ideally, the uterus should be removed to save the life of the patient in this situation. But this was her first child, if her uterus was removed, she would not be a mother any more. So, the doctor tried to normalize the uterine color by trying to press it with a hot mop. After the operation, the patient had to give 15-16 bags of blood in the ICU. For almost 2 months, the patient had to stay in the hospital. While leaving, husband and wife both conveyed unlimited gratitude to the doctor.

After some days, the couple came again to the doctor and said, "Please give me the medicine for having a baby".

The condition of the uterus was like that it had a lower possibility of child bearing. Even so the doctor gave some supporting medicines. During leaving, she said, "I know that I will conceive with your treatment."

I do not know any news further. Today I have caught sight of that woman after many days in the market. I heard that she had two children. The lady requested to pray
for her children.

I said, "Surely".

Key Message:
Regular health check up during pregnancy and delivering by skilled birth attendant reduces the risk of complication.

11. Life Stories

Amena was admitted to the hospital during her nine months pregnancy, with pervaginal bleeding.

In ultrasonography, it was found that the central placenta previa covered the opening of the uterus. Surgery was performed after collecting blood for transfusion.

The patient had a daughter of ten years old. Her husband was a simple man of the village. Before the operation, her husband said, "Madam, this is my only daughter. Please take care of her mother". There was an innocent softness on the big two eyes of the girl. Although the operation was quite complicated, the operation was completed by saving the uterus.

Time was about 11 pm, at night. A male baby was born and both of father and daughter were very happy. The doctor could not be as happy as the bleeding can start again at any moment. So, all necessary preparations were made as an emergency basis to combat the bleeding.

At three o'clock at night, the patient started uncontrolled vaginal bleeding. Then the uterus was removed by surgery. As far as possible precautionary measures were taken so that bleeding did not occur again.

After two hours internal bleeding was noticed again. The doctor felt helpless, what else would she do? There was nothing left to do.

The doctor looked at the girl and her father before entering the Operation Theater again.

The man said, "Madam, you put on your hand upon my little girl's head and pray a little. I know her mother will be cured".

The doctor's eyes filled with tears.

The operation was done again. After hysterectomy operation, two vault levels were absolutely cleared and bleeding came from there. After stitching those two layers, bleeding was stopped.

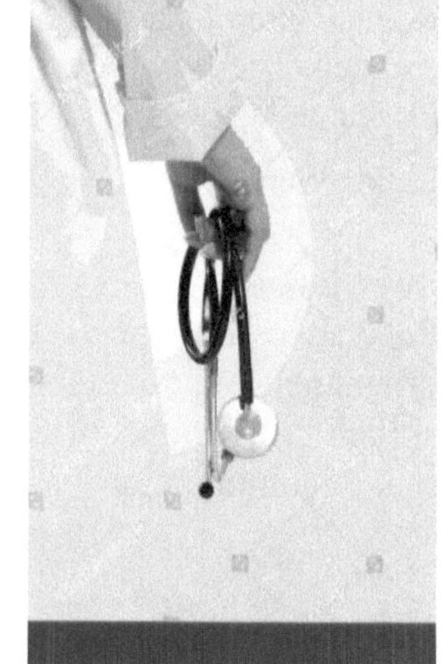

The doctor came out from the operation theater and told the girl, "Your mother has survived". Her smile made the doctor's attempts of whole night fruitful.

It is the success of the physician's life.

12. Life Stories

The house of Shampa's father-in-law was in a small city, Naogaon. After two years of marriage, there was no child; the mother-in-law was repeatedly asking for taking the baby. When Shampa said that they were trying to have a child, then mother-in-law had been silent. She guessed that as they were trying to take a child, one day they would be successful. There was no discussion any more at the father-in-law's house.

All members of their family were excellent and understood each other's pain. Considering probable pain of the couple, certainly nobody raised any question further anytime. However, the mother-in-law often asked for visiting a doctor.

They started treatment by a doctor in their home city. He prescribed medicine for a long time with no fruitful result. The doctor did not take any test of her husband Rasel.

After some treatment they lost their spirits, sitting quiet for a few more days. Then, according to the advice of another doctor, they came to the capital city, Dhaka to visit the new doctor.

In Dhaka, after ten years of marriage, Rasel was tested firstly. The doctor herein did not start any treatment without the husband's semen test.

Early in the course of Shampa's treatment, Rasel often had arisen this question that the child was born in joint participation of husband and wife. He might have any problem. Was there no need for any test or treatment for him? But again he thought if it was needed, the doctor would surely have told him. The doctor just mentioned it just after passing out of ten years.

They both went together to collect the report. Shampa was also given some tests. They went to the doctor's chamber with the reports. Both of them were skeptical, did not know, what bad news could be heard?

The doctor informed in depressive mode that there was no sperm in husband's semen. However, the result of the hormone was satisfactory. She hoped that enough sperm could be found in the testis although there was no sperm in semen.

Why such happened?

Rasel asked the doctor with anxiety, fear, helplessness and deprivation. The doctor informd that Rasel's two sperm duct were absent and it was a congenital defect. In some cases, two ducts might be closed due to infection or inflammation. In these cases, the sperm could be produced regularly, but the sperm could not come out because of blockages.

Rasel was silent on hearing this. Realizing his grief, Shampa said, "There is nothing to worry about, and is not it? Do not you have the treatment for this?"

Doctor informed that it is possible to have a child through the treatment of an advanced technology called ICSI. Both of them agreed for the treatment.

Their family members were informed of the matter. They did not hesitate to inform. Although Rasel's mind felt a little sad, he realized that it was his defect by birth. He himself was not responsible for it. So there was no reason to be inconvenienced. All family members encouraged them for a test tube baby by treatment. Knowing that expensive treatment and could not be successful at once, they began to treat themselves spontaneously. That spontaneity and support of everyone made them successful.

Key Message:
If a couple fails for child bearing inspite of trying, living together for one year continuously, they need to consult with physician.

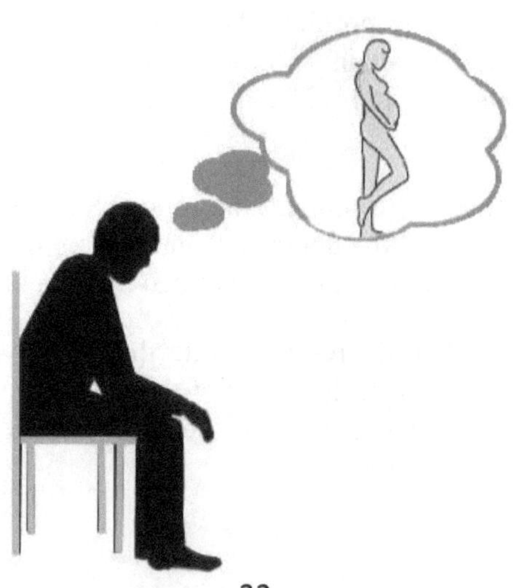

13. Life Stories

"My eldest son's fate may not bless him to see any child. So many people marry twice. What happens if he marries another for the sake of expansion of the family? "

Sharmin's daily routine became disgusting of hearing such from her father-in-law's house. Husband Ujjal did not care about the mother's words. He consoled Sharmin not to get hurt in any word of his mother.

They liked each other and got married. So, there was no shortage of understanding between them. Ujjal knows that the child is not conceived due to his physical problem. Of knowing this, he never tried to save Sharmin from his mother's words. Rather, he had always requested her not to share the issue of his physical problems with others.

They knew there were treatments for their problems. However, there was no IVF treatment facility in the country at that time. The treatment was multifold expensive in abroad. It was not possible for them. Both of them took their life easily.

But the day after day Sharmin was being poisoned by the words of her mother-in-law. Sharmin could not think of her life except Ujjal. It was also not possible for her to leave failing to cope with the torture of the mother-in-law. So, she requested Ujjal to inform the matter to her mother-in-law.

At last, he explained the matter to the mother and said that Sharmin had no physical problem. The factor for not having a child was Ujjal. The mother did not want to believe anyhow. Her confusion was that the males could not have such a problem. The responsibility was of the wife for being infertile.

Understading the limitation of the son she started giving more painful behavior towards Sharmin to cover up his fault. When she met someone, she started to talk in advance, "My eldest son will not see the child's face. What is the benefit of this sterile wife?" Ujjal was angry with mother's behavior. But the mother was not to be abandoned. So, he had nothing rather than to ask for forgiveness to Sharmin.

In the meantime, Sharmin's brother-in-law Utpol became father of a baby. For that happiness the mother-in-law used to provoke Sharmin as much as she can. Sharmin's days were passed in such a way.

Key Message:
Incase of infertility 50 percent male and 50 percent female partners are responsible. Expressing empathy towards the childless couple is our moral responsibility.

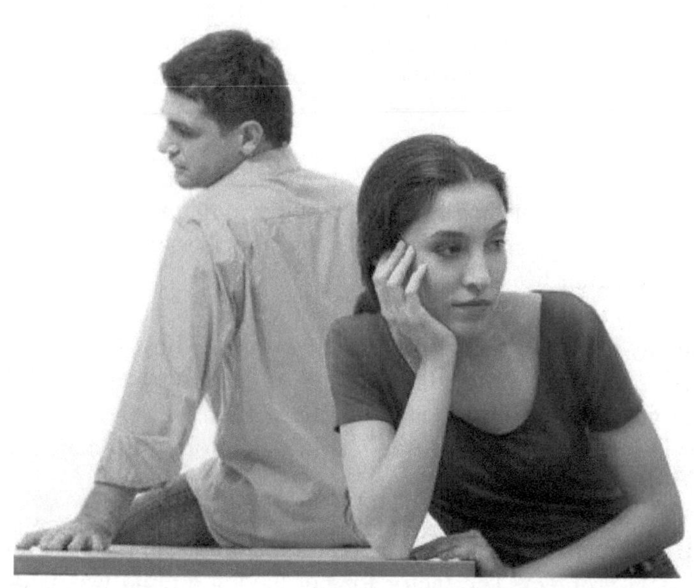

14. Life Stories

Umme Kulsum, almost forty three years old, took admission in the hospital ward. She was suffering from abortion at five months of pregnancy with complications. There were profuse vaginal bleeding and fever with shivering in the house. They did not want to express the correct history. But for medical treatment, it was necessary to have the right history. So, all the facts were known following a strategy.

Umme Kulsum had five children before. Husband plied rickshaw. The family was needy. She did not want child anymore. But they did not take any family planning method. Where to go to have these methods was also unknown to them.

Umme Kulsum consulted with a neighboring woman. The woman took her to an illiterate traditional midwife. She tried to make abortion through a 'Plant root medicine' inserting into the uterus. After two days, she had high fever with convulsion and started per vaginal bleeding, lower abdominal pain. Gradually the bleeding increased in amount. Two or three days passed in this way. Something like a fleshy mass got out but the bleeding did not stop anymore.

They came to the hospital due to rapid deterioration in the patient's condition. Immediate emergency treatment was started. Diagnosis was 'Septic abortion'. Treatment was given with antibiotics and blood transfusion.Only after passing six to seven hours, the patient was found being unable to eat anything, the jaw had become stuck. It was understood that she developed tetanus. At once the patient was referred to the 'Infectious Disease hospital' for treatment of tetanus.

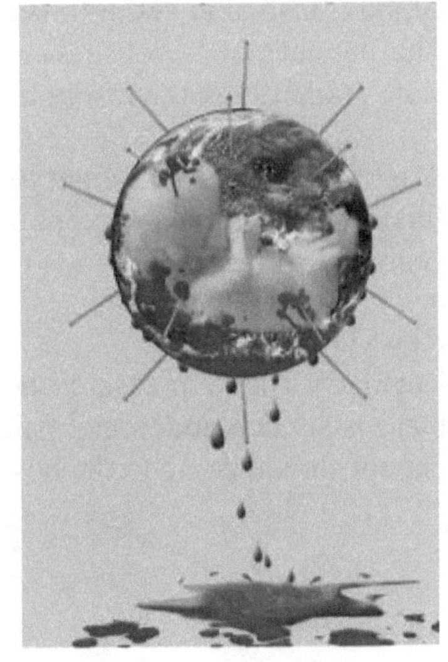

But in that hospital staying two days of inhuman sufferings, Umme Kulsum breathed her last leaving five minor children.

Key Mesage:
Adoption of regular birth control method is necessary to prevent unsafe abortion. For special needs, abortion can be performed under the supervision of a physician.

15. Life Stories

A patient was lying on the trolley. Doctor and nurse were offering intravenous saline to the patient.

The patient was unconcious. Teeth stuck with teeth with little bleeding cutting the tongue, fast pulse rate, and high blood pressure. A middle aged woman was standing next to the patient, the relative of the patient.

She reported, the patient had convulsion twice in the house. Full term pregnant. Her abdomen was felt abnormally hard and the heart rate of the baby could not be heard. The urine test showed that there was enough protein going out. It meant that the patient had 'Eclampsia' and possibly placenta was detached from the uterus causing bleeding inside, which is termed as "Accidental hemorrhage".

As the placenta was detached so the baby was endangered. The patient's relatives further said, about 24 hours before the patient's water bag inside the womb ruptured. As a whole, the patient's physical condition was complicated.

As a last effort to save the patient, caesarean operation was performed. The dead baby was delivered. It was appeared that the baby had died a few moments ago. When the baby was taken out, doctor found that the placenta was completely detached from the uterus. Blood was clotted just behind the placenta. Surgical procedures were completed fast. Blood transfusion and intravenous saline were being given in the body. The patient's consciousness still did not return. Finally, arrangements were made to run the respiration by artificial means.

After two days of fatal fight between death and life she failed to survive finally. By failing everyone's efforts she breathed her last leaving 3 years old son forever.

Key Message:
Regularly blood pressure should be measured during pregnancy. If there is sudden abdominal pain and vaginal bleeding during pregnancy patient should come to the hospital immediately.

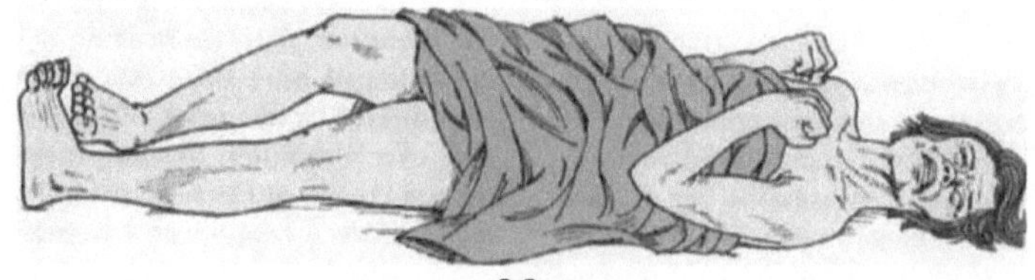

16. Life Stories

Razia was pregnant for the third time that year. During five months of pregnancy, the doctor recommended for some laboratory tests and ultra sonograph. Both husband and wife said, "Madam we do not want to perform ultrasound test anymore. In the last two pregnancies, ultrasonography showed child with congenital defects. Who knows what happens this time."

Razia's eyes were tearful. She started to weep saying, "My day night don't pass as usual after knowing the existence of a defective child in my womb. I cannot explain the scores of pain inside."

It was running four years after the marriage of Razia with her maternal cousin. At first both of them were in love and then they got married.

When Razia's first child was nine months in the womb she felt that the movement of the child was very slow. So, she came to visit the doctor. The baby's heart beat was not felt well. She was adviced to do an ultrasonogram. In the ultrasound report, the child found dead having developmental defects. Inspite of trying heart and soul to hide the matter to Razia, she understood that the child was no longer alive. Afterward all the arrangements were made for the normal vaginal delivery of the dead child.

After two days, she gave birth to a dead child. The new born child was examined and found several defects by birth, which could be easily traced by the naked eye. The mother was not shown the dead child as family members thought that the mother could be shocked by seeing the defective child and this memory could chase depression through out her life.

After two days the patient was discharged. The patient was advised to take Folic Acid, so that the next pregnancy decreases the possibility of congenital defects. Some tests were done to find out the cause of congenital defects. Nothing special was found. Razia and her husband returned home with the broken heart and empty lap.

After one year Razia couple came to the doctor again. This time the baby was about six months old inside the uterus and unfortunately the child's congenital defect was visualized in the ultrasound. Most of the educated patients are able to read the report themselves and understand what has happened.

There was no language to console her, and the doctor remained silent sometime. The baby survived for several hours after delivering. Some tests had been conducted for that time. Genetic counseling was arranged. The birth of a child with congenital defects twice was more likely to occur to the couple for the third time.

For the third time, Razia was no longer pressed to do ultrasonogram during pregnancy. Razia said, "I do not have any benefit in testing. Whatever has to happen, it is already there". Razia came again in the sixth month of pregnancy with a complaint of pervaginal bleeding and lower abdominal pain. That time Razia had a spontaneous abortion.

Razia's husband said, "I do not want to see the baby, just say whether it was a normal child." It was very difficult for the doctor to say that the child was born again with congenital defects. Finally, the doctor advised to adopt a child and bring up the child as their own child and teach well.

After few days Razia came back to the doctor and said, "I want to try to conceive a child again. As if a child is born, if it does not live then I'll adopt a child. No one can identify the child as adopted. It will be accepted as my own child in the society."

Key message:
Marriage between close relatives can often causes congenitally abnormal children for which prior planning and investigation are very important.

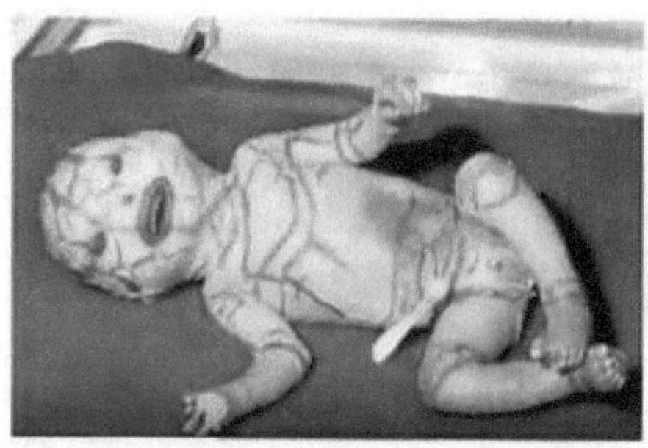

17. Life Stories

Chandrabati was very unhappy, sitting with a gloomy face. Her mother was worried. She had been sent to her mother's home from father-in-law's house with an ultimatum to return back with a healthy child.

Chandrabati's Blood Group was 'B Negative'. Just four days before she was admitted to the hospital with 36 weeks of pregnancy. The baby of the womb was smaller in size and had less amniotic fluid. The heart rate of the child was unusual. Without emergency delivery, the baby could not be saved. So, Caesarean operation was done to deliver the baby early.

During the operation, it was found that the water inside the womb was golden in color. The baby was pale and could not breathe naturally just after the birth. Exchange transfusion was arranged to change the blood. But the baby died within two hours after birth. There was no chance to change blood.

Chandrabati was married at an early age. She became pregnant one year after her onset of menstruation. She was not in an age to realize her own right or wrong. However, she remembered, she suffered from eclampsia (a convulsive disease during pregnancy) and later she gave birth to a dead child. Almost two years later, she gave birth to a son. That boy was alive.

She became pregnant once again before the year ended and gave birth to a dead baby at home at 36 weeks of her pregnancy. After almost two years, at 35 weeks of pregnancy, she gave birth to a dead baby again at home. Her heart was broken. Happiness in the family disappeared. For giving birth to dead children Chandrabati had to face humiliations defining her as a 'Witch'.

Her life had become miserable. This time she became pregnant for the 5th time, it was for the first time, she got opportunity to visit a doctor. The doctor tested the blood group and Rh factor and found that Chandrabati's Blood group was B and Rh factor was 'Negative'. Husband's Blood group was O and Rh factor was 'Positive'.

Since Chandrabati's blood group was negative and husband's was positive, the children of the womb especially the dead children possibly was containing positive blood for which they met the accident.

The scientific explanation is that if a mother with negative blood group bears a child in the womb with positive blood group and when the child is born, then its positive blood enters into mother's blood. The child's positive blood reacts with the negative blood of the mother's body. As a result, antibody in mother's blood is formed. The next time whenever the baby of the positive group comes into the womb, this antibody enters into the fetus's blood and reacts with the blood of the fetus. The blood corpuscles of the baby's body break down.

The more blood cells of the baby shall be broken leading to anaemia, making the body yellow due to jaundice, and swelling of the whole body with water and as a result, the heart will fail and baby will die. If the baby doesn't die, the child may be born with anaemia and jaundice or is affected by jaundice within twenty four hours of birth. It is difficult to keep the baby alive if it is not possible to change the blood of baby within a short time. The consequences depend on the amount of blood cell that was broken by Rh antibodies of the mother's body.

If the mother and the baby of the womb are Rh negative, then both the mother and the baby will not respond to anyone's blood due to same Rh negative factor. Most of the time it is seen that the first child survives from the affects of Rh incompatibility or reactions but it has an effect on the baby in next pregnancy.

The reason for the death of Chandrabati's first child was probably different. At that time, she had Eclampsia. The second child was alive, but the third and fourth child was born dead. The fifth or last was born in half dead and died within two hours of birth. Her children had been haunted in Rh incompatibility and died.

The first child and every subsequent child should be checked up the blood group just after the birth. If it would be positive blood group, then it was recommended for Chandrabati to inject Anti-D Gamma Globulin injection. As a result, antibodies would not be formed in the body of the mother; then other children born later would not be affected in uterus.

If Chandravati became pregnant later on, she should have checkup under an Obstetrician.

Key Message:

If mother's blood group is negative and newborn baby's blood group is positive, then mother should be given Anti-D Gamma Globulin injection within 72 hours of child birth.

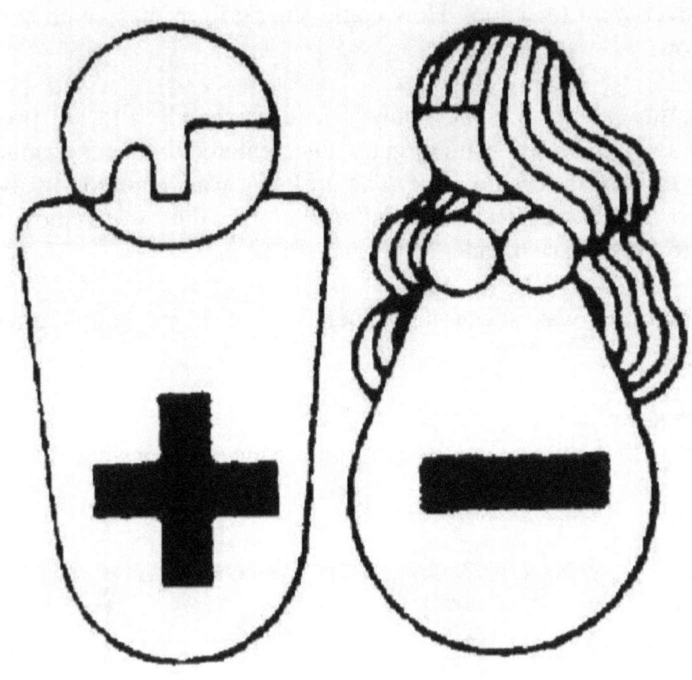

18. Life Stories

Shefali was 26 years old, light thin, sad face, unmarried.

Since birth, she had been suffering from continuous flow of urine. The girl was prisoned in a sad dark life. She grew up with no companion. She could not make any friend. She could not play with anyone, she never ever went to school. How could she perform these with constant urination?

The nature alone was her only friend in lonely life. It was her congenital defect, an extra urinary duct entered into her vagina. So there was no way to hold urine. The urologist was required to solve the problem. By the surgical intervention the extra duct was removed and added to the urinary bladder as normal situation.

The operation was successful. Shefali went home sound after the surgery.

Key message:
Consult with the physician for constant escape of urine since birth.

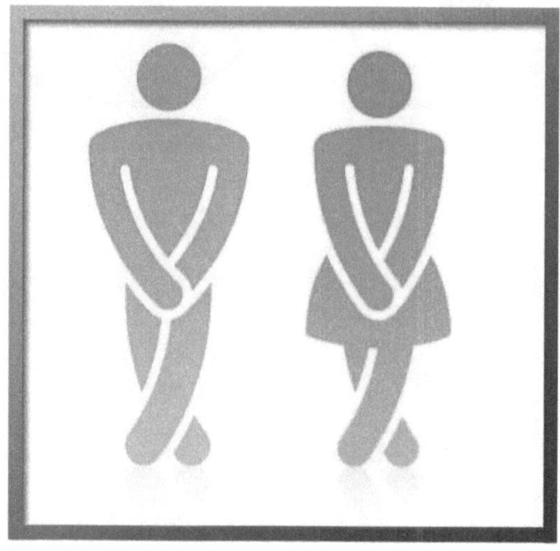

19. Life Stories

The doctors and nurses were in a high fume with the husband of a pregnant woman in the hospital.

The patient's husband said, "It is written in your discharge certificate that I had a healthy baby girl born. Where is that girl child?" The doctor and nurse said, "We have returned it to your wife's lap." The conversation was going on. After that, we knew the incident as follows:

Fatema Begum gave birth to the fourth daughter at this time. After hearing the cry of her new born female baby, Fatema just burst into tears. She said, "My husband will divorce me, if I go with this girl child, I will not be allowed to stay there; I'll be ousted'. I don't know what will happen to the fate of my existing daughters Sorna, Rupa and Mukta. I want to go back to them. Save my family, save my daughters lives."

The fact drew the sympathy of a nurse. She said, "I have a relative, and their financial condition is very good. They are educated, have been married for 10 years but they have no child, if you give the baby to them, they will bring up the girl very well."

In the end, there was a secret deal between them. The mother handed over the child in their hands.

The mother of a just born baby ornamented a story. She told her family members, "I've given birth a dead boy, it was a difficult labour, doctors performed a surgery to save me, cutting out the baby into pieces , so they have not shown me the dead body of the child. I also did not want to see."

Meanwhile, the doctor had given discharge certificate as a healthy girl was born. Mother and child were sound. The mother returned home crying.

Two days after going home, the husband and the family's people suspected for any reason, so they came to ask for the healthy daughter returned.

In collaboration with the hospital authorities along with mother's confession the child was brought back from the childless couple and handed over to the family.

Key Message:

A woman is not, at all, responsible for the birth of a girl child. The child will be a boy or a girl, is determined by the sperm of the father of the child. In this case, it is wrong to punish the mother for giving birth to a girl child.

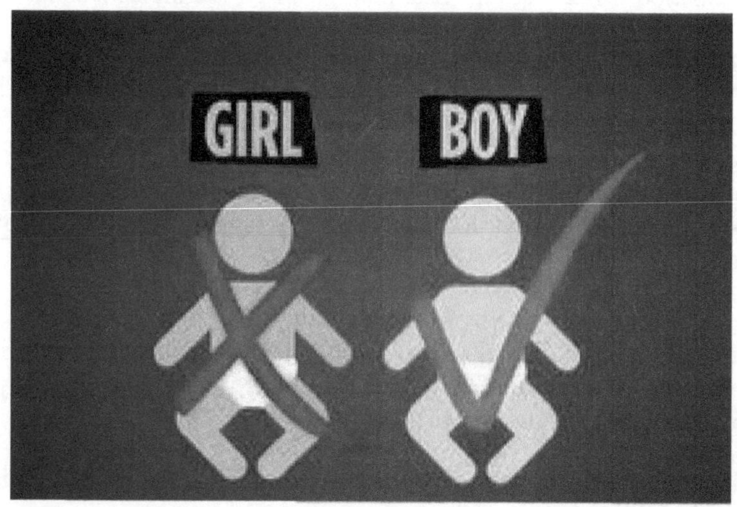

20. Life Stories

Zaynab Bibi was almost 52 years old. Menstruation had been stopped two to three years ago; again menstrual bleeding restarted few months back. She was taken to a different room for physical examination. When she was approached to examine internally, she was refusing for possible pain. It was found that urine flow was coming out through the vaginal canal. So, doctor decided to examine her under anaesthesia.

On examination, it was found that her urinary bladder was joined with the vagina by a fistula and there was a tumor in the opening of the uterus. Bleeding started when the tumour was touched. A portion of the tumour was dissected and the biopsy was sent for the histopathological test.

In the conversation with Zainab Bibi, the doctor asked, "You have not reported us of your continuous passage of urine."

Zainab said with long breath, "It was a history of thirty years. I was not willing to remember that. I had labour pain for two to three days when my first child was born. Three days later I was brought to the hospital. I was then unconcious. The baby was found dead in side the womb". She was silent for a while.

The doctor asked, "When did the continuous flow of urine start?"

Zainab said, "After almost a week of delivery, the bed started to be wet. I then came back to my father's house. My father and brother spent a lot of money. The specialist doctor was consulted, the doctor adviced to undergo to surgical remedy. But finally it was not done anymore. My husband divorced me."

Remaining silent for a while she said, "I was very pretty in my young life, after getting divorce, I got a lot of marriage proposals. I did not agree. I knew my marriage would not last long. I did not let others to know about my physical defects. Finally, a businessman annoyed me a lot to marry him. I agreed thinking something which I didn't know specifically. It was his second marriage who provided me with family maintenance support.

I had to maintain conjugal life with a lot of intelligence. I did not let anybody to understand that I had a big flaw. When he could detect the fault then after two or three years, he also divorced me. Where would my father and brother detach me, so I was with them till then?"

The doctor asked, "You must have had a bad smelled per vaginal white discharge before the per vaginal bleeding restarted. Why did not you come at that time?"

Zaynab said, "I thought of it as urine, so I did not pay heed to it. I was scared to see the bleeding. So I had come to you."

Zaynab Bibi came to the hospital but it was too late. Biopsy report showed cancer in the opening of the uterus. Cervical cancer was in such a stage that there was no scope to undergo a surgery. Finally, she was referred to the cancer hospital for radiotherapy.

Key Message:
In order to ensure safe delivery, delivery to be performed by skilled, trained, licensed midwife at the health center or at home. After three years of marriage, every woman should undergo the screening test for early detection of cervical cancer regularly. Cervical cancer can be cured if it is diagnosed at an early stage.

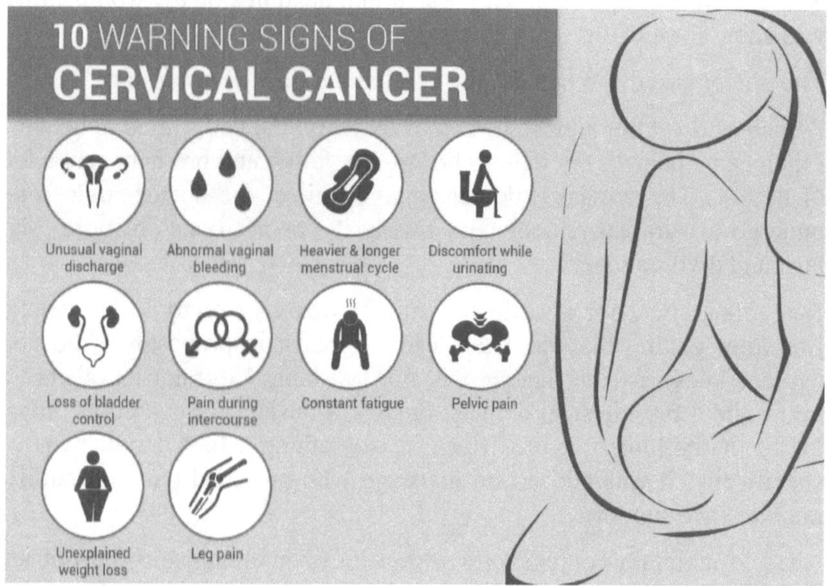

21. Life Stories

A father came to the doctor with his daughter of twenty-three years old, named Swapna.

The father said, "I arranged her marriage when she was 13 years old. She has been maintaining her husband's family for ten years. She does not have children. Earlier her husband arranged some medical treatment for her. Now the husband is not interested to spend for her. The son-in-law is thinking of getting married again."

Swapna did not say anything, her father was speaking alone. It seemed as if Swapna had kept the pain suppressed in her chest. She listened to her father's word with attention.

Both patience and money would be needed for the treatment. The father said, "Complete the treatment in low cost."

The doctor said, "What is needed to conceive a child, nothing more than that will be done. What is the benefit of only giving a nominal treatment, if no results are achieved? How far is your education done?"

Swapna's father replied," I let her married at the age of 13, where is the scope of education? "

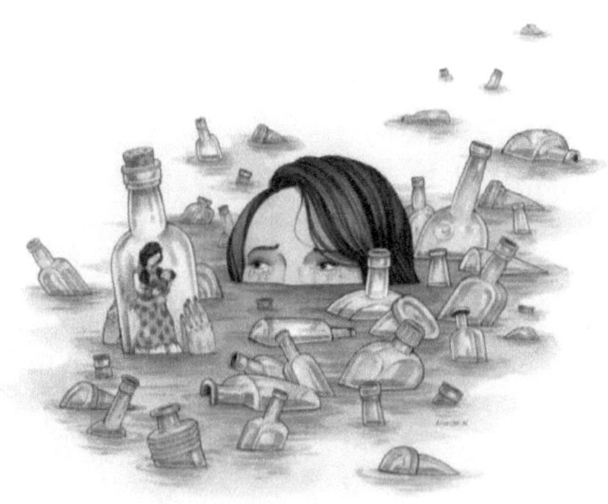

The doctor understood that Swapna was now a burden to the father-in-law's house as well as in her father's house. She needed to depend upon anyone or someone for the rest of her life. Many of the ladies didnot get married at her present age. After the physical examination, the doctor advised for some laboratory investigations and asked to meet with the reports.

While leaving, two eyes of Swapna were tearful. After a while she spoke. She said, "Who doesn't have any child, doesn't have any value in the society. I am a burden to everyone now. If I could stand on my own feet, then my trouble would have been lessened. It is very hard for anyone to be a burden. I am struggling with a lot of difficulties. Do whatever people say... Talisman, blessed water, grinded creeper leaves etc which I donot want to take, at all. Although I have no formal education but I'm able to understand that these are not actually the recognized treatment. But despite that I respect the beliefs of others to follow all.

The doctor said, "Wipe your eyes. I'm to treat you, let's see what happens."

Key Message:
Both husband and wife can be responsible for the inability to conceive a baby. It is not right to blame the wife alone. The early marriage should be stopped. Let every girl child be educated with a suitable education and transform into resource of possibility for family, society and the state.

22. Life Stories

Ramiza Begum, about thirty five years old, was lying on the operation table. She said holding the doctor's hand, "Stay with me. Do not leave me. Shall I survive if I undergo to surgical procedure? Shall I be able to go back to my sons?"

The doctor said, "Trust in Allah. Continue praying."

Ramiza Begum admitted to the hospital a few days ago. Her husband was a day labor. They maintained life from hand to mouth. There were three sons in their family. The eldest boy was ten and younger was six years old. It was quite normal to suffer from malnutrition. There was a big swelling in Ramiza's lower abdomen and it was painful for last two months. Her body was very weak, malnourished and under weight.

Almost two years ago she felt a small lump in her lower abdomen. The lump was moving from one side to another, she thought that there may be baby in the abdomen. The time was passing on and on. They could not understand what to do. They did not realize that it was required to consult with the doctor and treat accordingly. As there was no pain, they did not pay heed to it.

Since the past two months when pain started, they decided to go to the doctor. Who would take her to the doctor or to the hospital? The husband had to go to work to earn his daily income; otherwise they had to starve on the next day. Every day, every month and year would be continued in such a way of a day labor. Due to acute emergency her husband took her to the hospital, leaving his duty.

On physical examination, the patient was found lean and thin with severe anaemia. The lump of the abdomen had become very big. Almost whole of the abdomen was full of tumour. There was some accumulation of fluid in the abdomen (ascites). The tumour might be originated from ovary, signs and symptoms were leading to the possibilities of cancer. It should be confirmed by histopathological test of taking biopsy during surgery. The next treatment depended on the report.

Her blood group was ' O positive'; they could collect only two bags of blood. Two units of blood were needed to be transfused prior to the surgery. The anaesthetist said, "If she is not given two more bags of blood during surgery, then it may be a risk to the patient's life." Thinking about the possible risk he did not want to give anaesthesia.

It was not possible to buy blood on behalf of the patient's husband. Two among the doctors were interested to donate blood. Ramiza was no longer alone, everyone was there beside her. Anaesthetist came forward. The operation was started.

There was no fat under her skin. Water color became yellow in side the abdomen. Tumour was trapped by the food tube. A tumour weighing about four kilograms was taken out. Ovarian Cancer?

The surgery was completed. But surgery was not the complete treatment of the patient. There was a need for chemotherapy or radiotherapy. Perhaps the cancer had spread far and wide. If Ramiza Begum's tumour would removed by surgery at an early stage then perhaps it would have been possible to recover completely through a small operation.

They felt the lump of the abdomen almost two years ago. Two years were a long period. Side by side of passing the time, the cancer cells spreaded not only in the ovaries but also in many areas of the body. Ramiza Begum's life span had become shortened.

It might not be possible to run expensive chemotherapy treatment on their behalf. The government hospital had some affordable medical treatment, even there the possibility to get treatment, was also uncertain.

Key Message:
If any lump is noticed anywhere of the body then consult with a doctor immediately. In order to screen the cervical and breast cancer at an early stage it is necessary to come to health center.

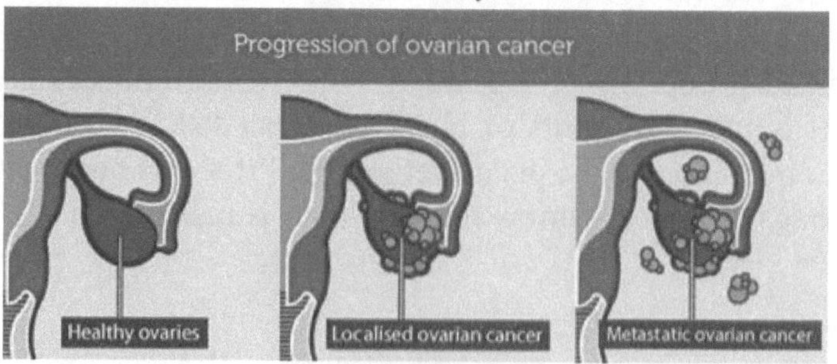

23. Life Stories

Doctor Aparajita, mother of three children had a mentally retarded child named 'Ontar'. While maintaining this child, she suffered from severe mental depression. Many times she wanted to quit the job. But everyone advised that the child might need huge money for the medical treatment. She had to deposit for the future of her child. So, the job was not resigned at last. Dr. Aparajita was performing her duties as well as maintaining the child.

There is a difference in the lifestyle between the Gynecologists than that of others. There is no night, no day, to be responded to emergency call. If the 'call' comes in mid night then disorder starts. All the sleepy people of the house are disturbed for openning and closing the doors of the home.

Last night Dr. Aparajitra received an emergency call. Her sick boy was sleeping. She was trying avoiding making sound inside the house. She silently came out of the house. Her husband closed the door. She went to the hospital by an ambulance. After two hours of heart and soul attempts, she could save the patient. While she was returning home it was half past 3 at night.

She came to the house and found that everyone in the whole house was asleep; she was thinking how would she call them? At first she called her husband. The agile man was tired and could not wake him. Then the other members of the house, even the domestic helping person were called; but no one heard the call of Aparajeeta. This half an hour seemed to be a long time for her. It seemed to her that she was the most helpless person in the world and was about to cry. Her tired body was not runnning further.

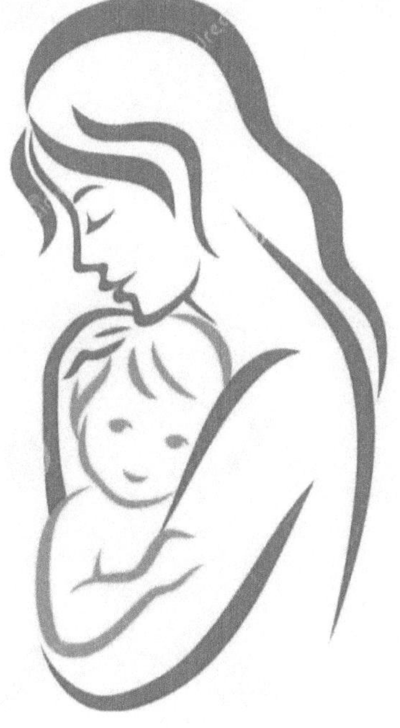

Despite the reluctance, she

wished to call him once!

"Ontar, my son..."

Instantly her son answered, "Yes mother."

Aparajeeta became upset. She wished to embrace her child in the chest. Tears filled her eyes. She said, "Call your father." There were seven members in the house, all were healthy and asleep. Nobody responded, but the disabled child was awake for the mother, when the mother would come.

The mother blessed her child for his long life.

24. Life Stories

Trishna is about twenty two or twenty three years old who came to visit the doctor with signs of night awaken depressive face. She was hesitating to talk for sometimes. When the doctor assured her, she started to talk in a low voice, "Madam, I got married at fifteen only. Afterward I delivered my first child. Immediately after that child, I gave birth to a boy who is now five years old.

I did a big mistake. Why did I trust? Why did I go with her?" The girl started to repent repeatedly.
The doctor said, "Tell me clearly, what happened? Where did you go and with whom?"

The girl started to say, "I studied in the same school with that girl. We didn't meet one other since a long time. When we met again she started to come to our house. I also used to share my story thinking her my friend of sorrows and happiness." She often said, "You are absolutely alone in house, husband is in office and children are in school, how do you pass time in home! A monotonous life it is."

One day she came to my house and told me, "You stay at home alone quite silently, let us go outside to visit anywhere. You'll feel well."

"The girl took me to a nice apartment. There were two youngmen there. They were talking quite gentle. After talking sometimes, I could understand that I fell into a trap. I wanted to leave again and again but they didnot let me to leave. My said lady friend left the room with one young man. I could understand that danger was imminent. I tried to go out but at last failed to do that. I was unable to shout due to shyness if neighboring people take it otherwise."

Keeping her silent for some moment she said in lower voice, "I was raped".

The doctor wanted to know whether there was a camera in the room.

The girl said, "I don't know. I'll not be able to share my pain with anybody. My husband will expel me from the house if he is able to know something about it. I'll not also get shelter in my parent's house. What shall I do? What will happen to my two children? How can I rectify my fault? What will happen to me if I become pregnant?"

The girl required to reduce her mental agony side by side with physical treatment on emergency basis. She needed counseling. The doctor advised, rendered medication and told to come for follow-up treatment. The girl stood slowly and left the room with heavy step.

Key Message:
Violence against women is a punishable crime. The victim requires at a same time physical treatment, mental support along with cooperation from law enforcing agencies.

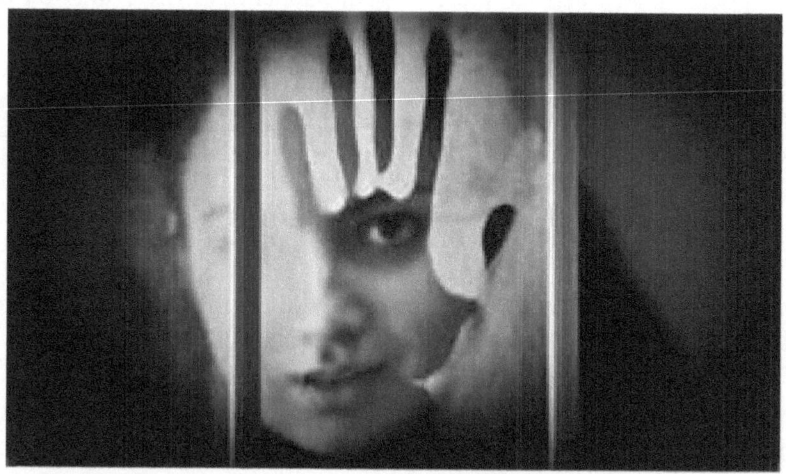

25. Life Stories

Mother and daughter covering with black-colored scarf came to the doctor. The mother said, "Please examine my daughter." The face was covered, only two eyes are visible.

The doctor asked the patient to lay on the bed for physical examination. She also said, "I will not be able to examine you if you do not open your face cover." The girl started to remove the face cover slowly.

From the eyebrows to forehead, the corner of eyes, and the cheeks all were burnt. It was understood that a terrible tragedy had happened in her life. The doctor asked, "How did it happen?"

The girl said, "Acid burn". Then she said the rest of the words herself.

"I was in class eight. My elder brother got married a few days ago. My brother's wife was very pretty. My brother had gone to town for work for a few days. I slept with my brother's wife at night. Suddenly, one day, at mid night something fell down on my face and body. All were burnt on my body. I started shouting.

Father Save me! Save me! Eyes and face were burning. Within a moment, everyone in the house woke up. I just heard that my father said, "Rinse water soon."

The girl stopped for a while. Then she began to say, "From then my physical, mental and family disasters started. I need to go to the doctors and to hospitals all the time. In the past 10 years, I have had plastic surgery for 13 times. What else can I say about that pain?"

"After this accident, I did not talk to anyone for four or five years, did not go to school. I did not like to read, I did not want to watch TV, nothing good about in this life."

"Many people came to talk with me sympathetically. One of them was the brother-in-law of my elder sister. I did not like him at all. He was a stubborn guy. He fell in love with me. I said that all of my body and mind was burnt. I had nothing to give. I had repeatedly rejected his love. But one day I also became weak to him due to his love appeal to me day after day." He said, "I want to marry you, I do not want your body; I love you and want you only". "Finally, I agreed to marry him in family pressure."

The doctor was going on to examine her listening to her. Gladly the doctor said that she has become pregnant since two months. Whenever the news was served to them, tears were rolling down from her mother's eyes.

The doctor asked, "Haven't your husband come with you?" The girl said 'No'. The doctor said, "I am eager to see your husband. Convey my salutation to him and say, madam wants to see you, wants to talk to you. When you will come later, bring your husband with you."

The mother and the girl left for home gladly. One month later, the girl came with her husband. The doctor examined her and could found that she was alright. The baby in her womb was growing properly. After seeing her husband, the doctor stood up and greeted him with Salam. The doctor said, "I saw a great man" The gentleman was very happy.

The girl was very fortunate. After such a big disaster in her life, she got a house, got the groom, got the family. Her family was going to be lighted with the arrival of a child who would be making them happy in the rest of her life.

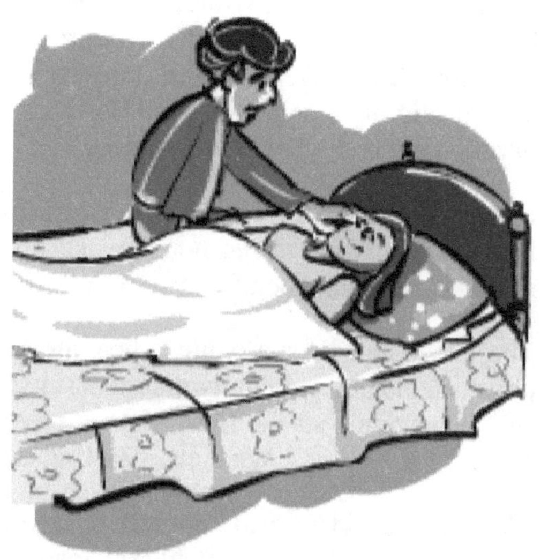

In this world, there is human evil spirit like the acid terrorists, at the same time; there are great men like her husband. That is why the world is still beautiful, habitable.

26. Life Stories

Razia was only 25 years old; educated.She was a primary school teacher, married to a businessman only one and a half years ago. She had a happy family.

For the first time she was going to be a mother. Her pregnancy care was done in a standard hospital. She followed the instructions of the doctors word by word to eat, drink, medicines, TT vaccinations etc. At the beginning of her pregnancy, she could not eat well due to anorexia, vomitting. After all, she was happy to take the taste of motherhood inspite of facing so much physical problems. Just after arriving at five months of pregnancy, she felt baby movement in her womb. The feeling of that day was very pleasant for her. Her preparations were increasing day by day, how she would welcome her child, take her to the chest, perform breast feeding... everything was working in her mind; she did not tell anything to anyone. The day of childbirth was approaching. Razia came to her mother's house.

From the evening her labour pain intensity was growing to higher scale. The pain was coming at a short interval. There was dark cloud outside in the sky. Thinking about the possible happenings, she trembled inside. She informed her mother. Her husband was not at home. She also told him over telephone regarding her future worries. She said to her husband, "All the arrangements are being made, don't worry about it."

A traditional birth attendant (TBA) was called. The little stormy air started to blow and at the same time, it was raining. Razia thought that her husband would have trouble to come in such weather.

Labour pain was frequently coming with little interval for whole night.There was storm outside. Everyone said, "It is to experience some pain to become a mother. We too have experienced such pain." Razia accepted their opinions.

At one time Razia said, "I'm unable to bear the pain now, take me to the hospital. Inform my husband." The news was also given to her husband. Razia's husband did not feel the need to stay with his wife during her crisis.

It was drizzling outside. Her relatives were thinking to take her to the hospital. The birth attendant told to bring pain increasing injection which would intensify the pain leading to deliver the child. The night was almost over and it was dawn then. The crows were crowing. The injection was injected to Razia to intensify the pain. It was felt that the womb was about to tear. Suddenly the cry of the newborn was heard and it was merged with Ajan of the Fazar prayer.

Razia was feeling absolutely happy. She had become a mother and asked to the TBA, "What is born dear?"

TBA said, "You've delivered a girl". Razia thanked God, but soon afterwards, she thought whether her husband and the people of her father-in-law's house would be happy or not.

After a while Razia felt that hot fluid was coming out of her uterus sponteneously. Everyone said, "It's normal."

Razia said, "I see all dark. I'm going to die."

Yes, so! All of her clothes were getting wet in blood.Razia's mother said, "Let's go to the hospital quickly." An auto rickshaw was called. She was lifted there; auto rickshaw became bloody.

Auto rickshaw puller said, "I will not take such patient." Another auto rickshaw was called. In this way, valuable moments for life were lost.

At the auto rickshaw, three passengers became completely blooded. They reached the hospital gate at 8:30 in the morning.

The doctor found her with a white pale face, cold body, rapid pulse; unmeasureable blood pressure. She was given intravenous saline, oxygen, and cardiac massage. But there was no response. The eyes had become fixed. After examining her, it was understood that the uterus was ruptured during the child was born and within two hours, all the blood of the body drained out.

And thus she lost her life in slow pace.

Key Message:
As a part of the pregnancy and delivery preparation arrangement should be done for transportation to hospital in case of emergency.If possible child should be delivered in the health center. It is not, at all, recommended to take any medicine from 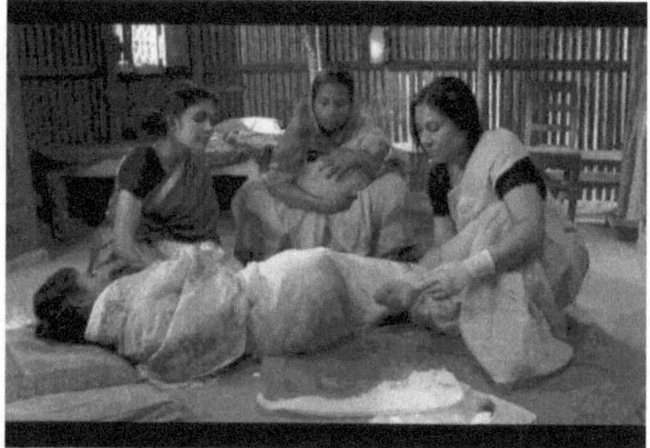 any unskilled TBA to increase labour pain. Above all, the husband's presence is very desirable in such a situation.

27. Life Stories

Hasina had been admitted to the hospital. The bed was flowing with her blood. She was having excessive per vaginal bleeding. All treatments to stop bleeding including intravenous fluid had been given. Nurses, doctors and others were working fast. Knowing the history from the husband he was sent to collect blood for transfusion. Without immediate blood transfusion patient could not be saved.

The mother of three children, Hasina gave birth to a new born by Caesarean section only 20 days back. Removing the stitches of surgery, she returned home well. The patient was again brought back to the hospital due to excess pervaginal bleeding.

After leaving the hospital, she had to do all the works of the family alone. Every husband should help her wife taking care of children and other house hold works. It did not happen in Hasina's life. She could not take rest after her delivery. They had single family, small children, and one of them was new one. Although she felt feverish but she did not pay heed to it. Taking the Paracetamol tablets had reduced fever. The body was maintaining in this way thinking that the weakness was probably due to her surgery. Her husband did not take the matter into consideration.

Suddenly there was discomfort in her abdomen. At first there was a little pain, after which per vaginal bleeding was started. Although initially it was small in amount but later on excessive bleeding was continuing. She realized that it should not be right to stay at home; something unusual was going to be happened. She was admitted to the hospital.
After receiving primary care Hasina opened her eyes, held the doctor's hand and said, "Please save me doctor, and don't delay as I'm feeling pain in my abdomen. Please perform the surgical remedy soon." The doctor also realized that she could not be recovered without surgery. The operation was started after collecting blood. After openning the abdomen doctor found that the site where the Caesarean section was done was infected and spreaded nearby blood vessels.

In total 9 bags of bloods were transfused to her. Within few weeks, Hasina became cured. The little boy was taken care keeping together with the mother. While returning home with smiling face, she expressed gratefulness to the doctors.

Key Message:

If fever develops within 40 days of delivery of a child then it should be taken into account. The mother needs sufficient rest and care. Husband and other family members need to cooperate to take care of the children. Family should be aware of this matter.

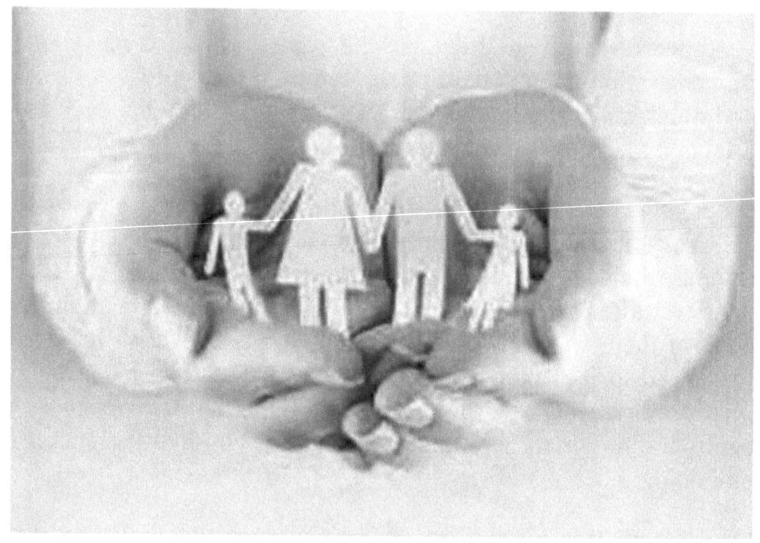

28. Life Stories

Ramija was of twenty four years. Her husband worked as a supervisor in a garments factory. Ramija had a five years old child. She was pregnant for second time. During her antenatal period she took tetanus vaccine only once. That was the only pregnancy care she received.

There was no problem during her previous pregnancy; delivery was performed in the home. The physical condition was not good from the beginning of this second pregnancy. First time, the delivery was performed at her mother's house; again she had come to her mother's house for second delivery.

During her last trimester of pregnancy, she developed leg swelling. For the past fifteen days, she was feeling unwell. Eyesight seemed to be slightly blurred with increased headache. They did not take the matter seriously. The husband was also unresponsive.

At five o'clock in the morning, coming back from the toilet she experienced severe pain in her abdomen with vomiting. She said, "Mother, it is not the labour pain. Do not know what is going to be happened?" Her eyes were overturned saying so. It started convulsion. She could not be kept on the lap.

Immediately her mother took her to the hospital by hiring an auto rickshaw. She had convulsions on the way to hospital for about five or six times.

The doctor examined her blood pressure which was too high. Eclampsia had a specific form of convulsion, it could be understood, that convulsions were caused by Eclampsia. I.V channels (quick blood vessel injection system) and catheter (urinary bladder evacuation arrangement) were performed as well as magnesium sulphate was injected in the vein and muscle. The baby's heart beat was falling downward rapidly. Immediately after primary management of convulsion, Caesarean operation was carried out.

The baby was delivered almost in a suffocative state. The newborn baby was sent to ICU for emergency management. Mother's bleeding began at the operation table. It began from all sides including the area of the incision, the uterus and the ureter. It was understood that due to eclampsia 'HELLP syndrome' had developed. 'Fresh Blood' was needed in such a situation. The first twenty four hours passed with 3 bags of blood transfusion. The patient was nearly unconscious for twenty-four hours. A doctor and a nurse were taking care of her.

One day after, the patient's condition improved. When she was called by her name, she opened her eyes and looked. Smile was on everyone's face. The whole night's fatigue went away. Ramija was trying to talk quietly.

Two days later, her condition improved. The baby was lying near her chest. The doctor asked, "Do you remember what happened during the convulsion period?" She said, "I had untolerable pain, I did not have any sense". The doctor said, "Can you now recognize us?"

She said, "Doctor, I could identify my mother and sister two days ago." The doctor said, "Now go home being cured"

After a few days, Ramija told the doctor with a nice baby on her lap in a smiling face, "Madam, I have been discharged with advice. Please bless my son."

The doctor said, "My blessings will be with you for all the time."

Key message:

Regular health check up during pregnancy, blood pressure monitoring and quick shifing to the hospital in emergency situations is essential to get healthy mother and baby.

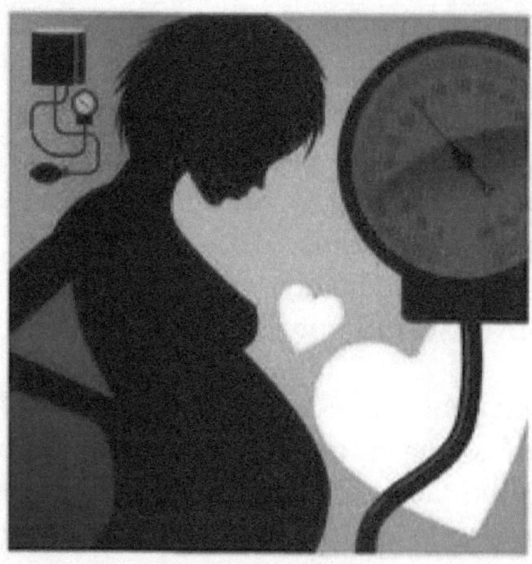

29. Life Stories

A medical technician came to the doctor and said, "Madam, my sister-in-law has been hospitalized. Nobody can identify the disease. Various investigations have been done. Will you please visit her?"

Entering into the cabin the doctor found a nice young lady was about to die. The patient was examined hearing the history from her relatives. It was assumed to be a lot of bleeding inside the patient's abdomen. Probably, her pregnancy was in the fallopian tube. As a result, the tube was raptured and bleeding occurred. In medical term it is called 'Ectopic pregnancy' which refers to implantation of fertilized ovam any site instead of appropriate place inside the uterus.

Although the patient had bilateral tubal ligation as permanent method of contraception but it was decided to undergo surgery. Sometimes the ligated tube itself can join automatically. Doctor said, "Sign in the consent letter for operative procedures, collect four bags of blood." Every moment was important for saving the patient's life.

The operation was started; the patient's abdomen was opened and found a huge amount of collected blood inside the abdomen. The ruptured fallopian tube was hold and tied well. Very easy operation but decision making was difficult. About four bags of blood had to give to the patient.

The patient was recovering quickly. But there was a panic on her face which faded her beauty. She was suffering from death phobia. The doctor advised to consult with a psychiatrist.

Key Message:

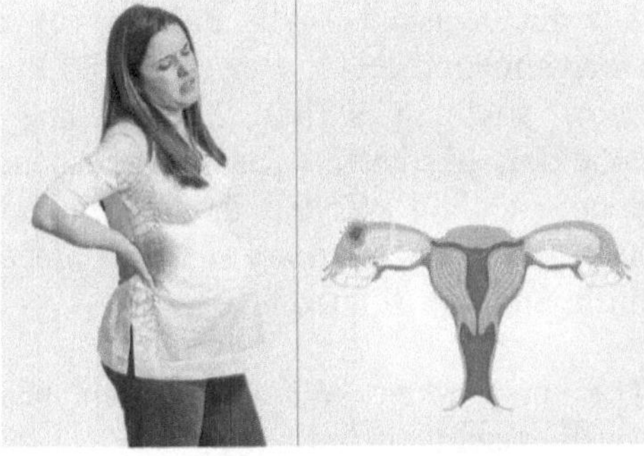

If any woman of reproductive age group experiences suspension of menstruation along with lower abdominal pain and slight per vaginal bleeding, then along with consideration of other possible diseases 'Ectopic Pregnancy' should be kept in mind. This is an emergency situation.

30. Life Stories

The patient was very lean and thin, pale appearance, lips and eyes were absolutely white. She was breathing fast. The pulse was rapid and weak, blood pressure also fell down. This was her sixth pregnancy. Just fifteen days ago; the patient gave birth to a low weight child which was delivered in home. Since then, her pervaginal bleeding was continuing more than normal level. When she was near to death, her husband brought her to the hospital. Diagnosis found 'Anaemic heart failure'' or anaemia induced heart failure.

The amount of haemoglobin in the blood had dropped to 4 grams, which was supposed to be at least 12 grams per liter. The x-ray of the chest showed enlarged heart and there was a sign of water accumulation in the lungs. Patient's heart needed special care. But it was not possible to shift the patient to specialized hospital without improving patient's general condition by providing first aid.

The patient was treated with oxygen in the semi sitting position and the accumulated fluid was taken out of lungs by the injection. Only one bag of blood could be arranged by the husband of the patient. Patient needed more blood. It was not possible to collect blood on behalf of her poor husband. The arrangement was done for withdrawing money from the 'Poor Fund' of the hospital. One doctor donated blood himself. One nurse and a doctor were assigned for continuous care for the patient.

The sister-in-law of the patient was just beside her.

The doctor asked, "Why did not you bring your patient before such worst situation?" Her answer was, "I live in another village. I could not know anything earlier. I did come quickly hearing her serious condition. My brother (patient's husband) had three little children. The youngest child was left in the neighboring house.The previous child had died in the abdomen and the immediate last one had died after the birth. She was ill fated."

The nurse asked "Why the patient bears the child inspite of having severe anaemia in her body?"

The patient's sister-in-law said, "When she was pregnant for three months they went to the doctor for abortion. Doctor said that before doing abortion she needed urgent blood transfusion; otherwise the mother would fall in life threatening situation. Then they did not proceed."

Doctor asked, "Where is the patient's husband?" She said, "Brother has gone to pull the rickshaw, how will he feed the children if he does not go to pull the rickshaw?"

The doctor said, "Bring 15 days old child of the patient to the hospital."

The patient's condition improved a lot in the next day. The child was under weight. Even the movement of the intestine of the baby was visible. The child had been suffering from sepsis, so the baby was admitted to the newborn ward. After two days, there was a little improvement in the condition of mother and child.

Then her husband was called and informed that the heart of his wife had become very weak due to severe anaemia. Her heart was unable to work properly. She needed treatment. She was being referred for specialized treatment in a heart hospital. She might need admission for treatment. Otherwise, the patient couldnot be saved. No more babies should be conceived. Follow birth control methods.

In fact, she would not get rest going back to the needy family. She had to do all the works in the family including taking care of the youngest child and three other children. There was none to help her there. As a result, pressure on her heart would increase, would be very weak and would proceed to final resting place leaving behind the four children and the family.

Key Message:
Let the birth of every child be preplanned. In order to prevent anaemia it is necessary to take green leafy vegetables and fruits.

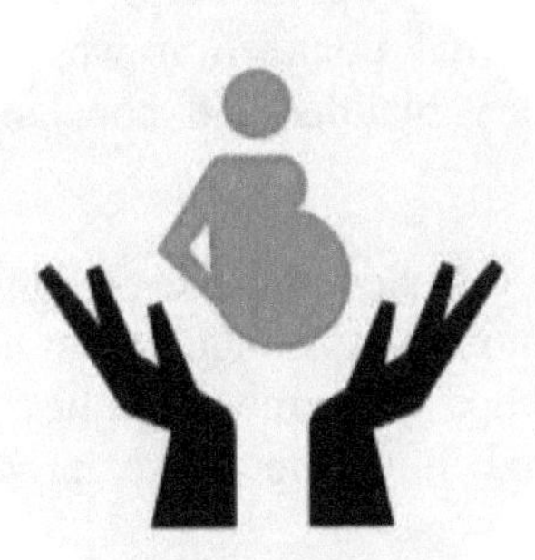

31. Life Stories

A lean and thin figured adolescent girl Rabeya (weighted 40 kg) was married only two years ago with a butcher of a meat shop. The father of Rabeya was a day labor and mother was involved with house hold works in the houses of other people. They simply maintained the family taking a small house on rent just to keep the body and soul together.

She became pregnant within two months of marriage. She could not have good food in the house of her father-in-law. The mother-in-law often used to oppress her. There were only mother-in-law and husband in the family. Her husband had never ever taken her to any health center for check up during pregnancy. The mother of Rabeya took her to the house of Rabeya's father when Rabeya was pregnant for five months. Since then, she lived with her mother. Her husband came and met every now and then.

The delivery date of the pregnant arrived. A birth attendant was called when labour pain was felt in full term. After her trial for one day to augment labour she told , "It is not possible for me, please take her to the hospital". Her husband left her in home keeping in such a condition and had not inquired further. In the mean time, one day passed to take decision to bring her to the hospital and to collect money. When two days crossed, then the land lord took her to the hospital and admitted her.

When she was brought to the hospital she was all but unconcious. After examining the patient, the doctor found that it was an obstructed labour. The baby in the womb died in suffocation. Surgical intervention was urgently needed otherwise the patient would die due to rupture uterus or later on Vesico Vaginal Fistula (VVF) would develop.

Dead baby was delivered by operative procedure. Doctor's prediction became true. An abnormal connection was developed between the vaginal wall and urinary bladder and constant escape of urine was started.

Discharging her from the hospital the patient was instructed to get admitted after three months to undergo to a surgical procedure so that the constant escape of urine may be stopped. Rabeya was fortunate as she cured after operative procedure. The operative procedure should be done by very skilled hand and accurately. Otherwise there is a possibility of failed surgery.

Rabeya went to her husband's home but he was unwilling to keep her at home. Rabeya asked her husband, "Could you leave me if my baby would survive? Pay at least for my livelihood maintenance cost and medical treatment."

No. She was not given anything. She returned home from hospital with an empty lap and with a big physical defect. Her husband's home returned her with an empty hand.

Key Message:
If Caesarean section could be performed within 12 hours of labour pain then Rabeya might not have faced such suffering. She could return home with a healthy new born baby. A nice family life…

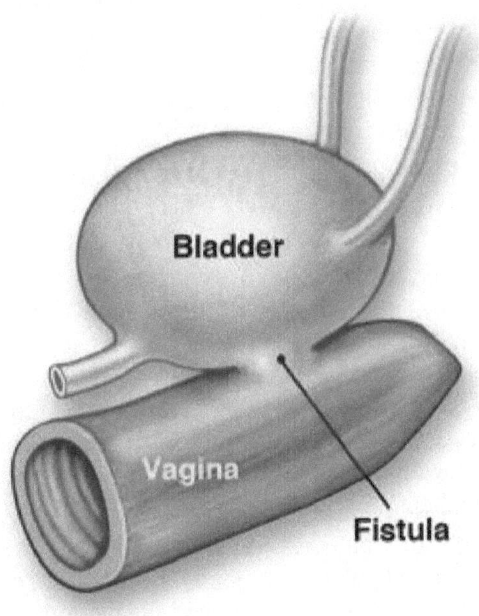

32. Life Stories

Yanur had become pregnant for the second time after a prolonged period of twelve years. Her first baby was born in home, still alive and read in a school. No antenatal check-up was done in the current pregnancy. She received only two doses of TT vaccine.

When labour pain started she told, "Please let me take to the hospital".

But the people of the home of the father-in-law's told her, "The delivery of daughter-in-law of our family is performed in home."

They at first brought a traditional birth attendent; she tried, but could not conduct the delivery. Then another traditional birth attendent was brought. She also was unsuccessful. The patient was suffering from severe pain. She again and again requested, "Now take me to the hospital, save my baby". But in vain, they then brought another traditional birth attendent.

Accordingly four traditional birth attendents attempted one by one for delivery. Each of the trials was very inhuman and unhygienic. One of them tied the abdomen tightly with light towel. Repeatedly examining the vagina she told, "See whether the hair of the baby is seen or not, if it is seen then I'll pull out the baby outside." Two persons held the legs pressing, one was pressing on the abdomen and another was pulling keeping hand inside the vagina.

Yanur tolerated all with a hope to see the face of a newborn baby. When all the traditional birth attendents were failed, then Yanur was almost in a dying condition and was admitted in emergency department of a hospital.

After examining her, doctor started to render the treatment by giving antibiotics and I/V saline. The pulse of the patient was fast but feeble, the blood pressure fell down; the heart beat of the baby in the womb had become abnormal. If Caesarean operation was not conducted, then the baby along with the mother would die. The condition of the patient was so critical that any accident may happen in operation table. The operation was conducted talking with the family members of the patient, receiving the 'Risk Bond' from them.

The lady gave birth to a baby. The child passed stool (Meconium) inside the uterus and also had eaten that stool. The stool had entered into the respiratory tract of the baby. The baby was unable to breath. Pediatrician was present at the operation theater. They were trying to clean the meconium from the respiratory tract of the baby and the baby was not able to cry.

All on a sudden, the baby started to breathe slowly. The newborn was treated with oxygen, I/V saline, antibiotics and heat.

Failing all the attempts of the doctors, the baby died after two hours.

On the other hand, the condition of the patient was at a stake. She was kept in the ICU. Oxygen, blood, suction and antibiotics all were applying at a time. But from the next day, her abdomen became distended. The sound of her intestine could not be heard. Different laboratory tests for diagnosis were continuing. At last after four or five days it was decided to perform operation again as the last attempt to save the patient.

When, it was asked for permission from the people of her father-in-law's house they instantly replied, "What will we do with her as we lost our baby?"

How inhuman behaviour is it! Then the sister of the patient came forward and told, "Doctor, please save my sister in any way you can." Considering the operative risk, operation was conducted taking 'Double Risk Bond'. It was found that huge pus was accumulated inside the abdomen and the uterus had become black, gangrenous.Infection was spreading from this uterus. After taking permission from the relatives of the patient, the uterus was removed.

The patient was discharged when she recovered. She left in empty lap and broken mind. Milk was still secreting from her breast, she would never be able to feed her baby. She would never ever have the experience of menstruation.

Her mental pressure was beyond the capacity to measure. The physicians had hold her life in any way; but she left hospital in all but in a dead state.

Key Message:

In order to give birth to a healthy baby and to restore the optimum health of the mother, delivery to be performed with skilled, trained up and license holder midwife. It is possible to reduce the risk of child birth by performing the delivery in a health center.

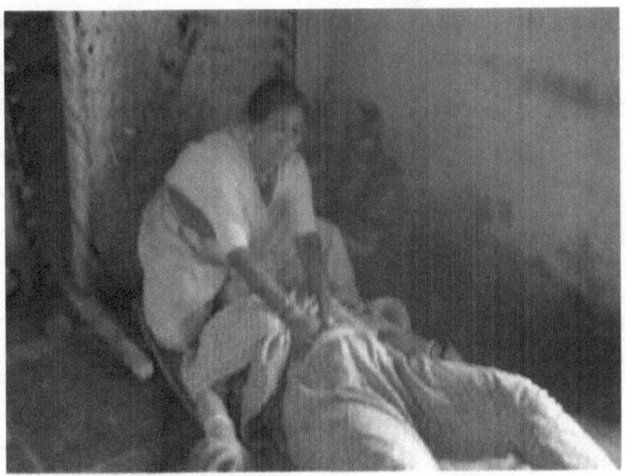

33. Life Stories

Bangladesh has achieved significant progress in the empowerment of women. The Prime Minister of the country, Leader of the opposition party, Speaker of the National Parliament, all of them are women. In our country, women represent 49.4% of the total population. But how much power really they hold at home and outside? As I'm a person involved in medical science, I have the opportunity to interact with women from different social classes and professions everyday. Here I'm sharing some of my experiences that I got while discussing with them, and treating them.

Perspective 01:

In the present scenario of the world, infertility has become quite prevalent. According to medical science, the reasons behind infertility are accounted as 50% due to men and 50% due to women. However, in our country, still the women are solely blamed for not having any child. In many cases, the male partner is responsible for infertility. But they don't believe it, or don't want to admit it. Some of them go for second marriage to save their lineage. But no child is born there.

Perspective 02:

The government provides free maternity service. Even though, 36% of the pregnant women don't obtain that service. Among them, a large portion thinks that they don't require that service. As the women are not financially independent, they cannot establish their rights and regular needs in the family. They don't have the authority to take decisions and thus they are even deprived from the healthcare services which are free. Though the government is encouraging to deliver child at the facility at free of cost, still now 62% of the child are born at their houses.

Though the screening of cervical cancer is done for free, in the last 12 years we could include only .4% of the total female population into the process.

62% of the couples are using birth control methods, and the decision of the male partner gets more priority here. How many children should they take, what birth control method should they use, these things are also decided by the male partner in the family.

Perspective 03:
According to Bangladesh Demographic and Health Survey [BDHS], child marriage rate of Bangladesh in 2014 was 59%. Taking the child daughter on his lap, the father may dream that one day his daughter will grow up and be in some respected job. Though the government provides free education, many of us cannot utilize this opportunity. Many feel insecured with a growing up daughter at house. It seems that their responsibility is fulfilled if they can arrange a bridegroom for her.

Perspective 04:
We don't have any proper and adequate discussion in the society regarding the issues like natural physical changes during puberty, arrangement during menstruation, the process of impregnation, the spreading and prevention of sexually transmitted diseases, etc. For these reasons, we find ignorance, superstitions and wrong explanations regarding these issues and the reproductive health of women is at risk today. As there is no opportunity for proper management during the period of menstruation, many of the girls remain absent in school during that time. If they remain absent for 3 to 4 days per month due to this reason, then in a year they'll be absent for 36 to 48 days. It affects their result in the exam, and their confidence.

The frequency of sexually transmitted disease in adolescent girls is increasing as they don't have any appropriate knowledge about the spreading and prevention of sexually transmitted diseases. They don't have complete knowledge about the process of impregnation. So, when they get pregnant, they choose the path of abortion. In most of the cases, it is done secretly, and following insecured method. Still at present, one of the major reasons for maternal death is unsafe abortion.

Perspective 05:

While passing through our life, our mental health is constantly afflicted by various illogical prohibition, negligence, injustice, torture and violence. According to the information of Bangladesh Maternal Mortality and Health Care Survey [BMMS] 2010, among the premature deaths of women, 9% is suicide, 14% is maternal, and 21% is cancer. But have we taken any initiative to prevent this 9% death due to suicide?

Perspective 06:

The homemaker in the family takes care of every need for every member in the family, including their fooding, clothing, medicine etc. She covers everybody with her blanket of care. But do the other members in the family look at her needs and requirements? Do they ever ask whether she's taking her medicine in proper time or not? As we're always coping up with these norms and customs, it seems that we women have forgotten how to ask what we need.

Perspective 07:

A few days ago, I went to an internationally renowned insurance company to insure an education policy for the future education life of my child. There I was informed that to do this, I need a written approval from my husband stating that he doesn't have any objection.I asked them, if my husband comes here for the policy, would he require my approval? Then I learned, no, it won't be required.

It will take some time for us to get out from this web of conventional ideology and practice, and establish freedom and equality for women in reality. We're now passing through a transition period. Though the society has achieved significant progress in education, information technology, and per capita income and so on, when we go back to our home after finishing our daily work, most of us look for that universal role of a woman that we have seen earlier, or have read in the novel. And when we don't find it, we get stumbled. People express it in different ways. If anybody wants to show any positive expression, it seems that the society is holding him back.

I believe that we cannot ensure women's right only by enacting laws. All the male and female of the society need to realize and accept it

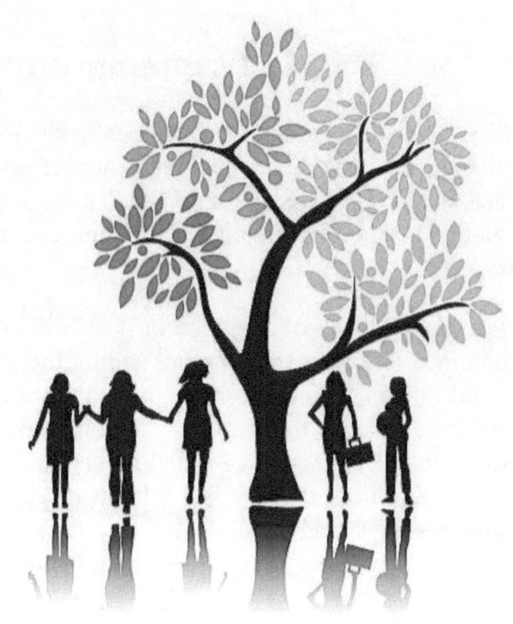

from their heart. We need to practice equality in our family, so that the future generation can learn from it. Otherwise the women in high positions will remain as mere ornaments of our society. The mass people will not get any benefit from it.

Let's change ourselves

"Egalitarianism of men and women in the journey of development will change the world, a new dimension to the work." Our women are hardworking, brave, and talented. Today we need a change of attitude on the question of equality. This change must start from the family and society.

Poverty and lack of social security still limit the parents of girl child to embrace child marriage before ending the school. The government has made access to free education, but on the way to reach school, who will give the security to the girl? Minimum age of marriage ought to be 16 or 18 there of no issue of social movements. We need to build a society where a girl can equally feel safe inside and outside the home. In many families investing in daughter's education, nutrition, health, and the cost of daily needs do not seem a lucrative investment than investing in son.

According to UNICEF; Bangladesh ranks fourth in the rate of child marriage in 2015. Sixty five (65) per cent female children of this country get married before eighteen (18) years. The girls who become pregnant before 18 years, experience adverse physical, mental effects for mother and baby too. These mothers are seldom able to play the role as an ideal mother in future.

Sometimes we hesitate to provide the necessary health information to the teen age girls during puberty. This leads to prejudice and misinterpretation. Grief-stricken reality is that misinterpretation among the adolescents now-a-days has more or less the same extent of misinterpretation which I experienced twenty five (25) years back.

The girls with a lot of physical inconveniences sometimes cannot tell her family or a teacher. That's why each health care center must have one (1) adolescent corner where they will be able to find solution to their problems freely.

Due to lack of family and social support, large number of girls opted to stay away from challenging profession. Some fracture to come in the middle of the boulevard. We need to increase the family and social support for the women. Husband should play an important role in this regard. Eighty (80) percent female of this country at some time in their life is abused by their husband.

Only two point one percent (2.1%) took legal action against it. Many rich, established women endured her husband's abuse due to lack of social security. The image is same in rural and urban areas. Very few women are able to swear that they have not heard anything disgraceful from her husband in their lifetime.

We should work to bestow women the opportunity to prove their ability, safety in workplace, freedom of movement, standard day care center to look after her child in absence of her. In Bangladesh, still there is inadequate day care center compared to the needs. According to the labor law, if there is forty percent (40%) of female worker in an institute, there should be day care facility for the children up to the age of 6. It is necessary to monitor its implementation. During office hour, many parents prefer to keep their child in day care center than to domestic workers.

The commendable role of Bangladesh is reducing maternal mortality rate. Sixty two (62) percent of mothers still give birth at home. Fifty six (56) percent give birth at the hands of the traditional birth attendent. That means by the persons who do not have any scientific training on this topic. Often they cannot determine the complicated condition inside the womb, during birth and postpartum, cannot take immediate necessary action. In spite of Government's free facilities, women's are not coming to the health centers for delivery due to poverty, religious and social bigotry and lack of awareness, lack of necessary vehicles or bad conditions of the road. Lack of female doctor or Caesarean section fear also works here. We should pay attention to these issues to achieve sustainable development.

Women across the world deserve a generous and respectful health care. What do we mean by respectful health care? While providing health care women should be given appropriate privacy which is a part of it. In our country doctors of busy public or private hospitals sometimes do not pay proper attention in this issue. Simultaneously 2/3 or more patients are giving history or physically examined. In front of many people/doctors when a woman is asked about her personal health problems, many women feel embarrassed and do not open up all the problems. Some of them stop consulting doctors to avoid this embarrassment. We will have to give every patient's privacy as her honor. Details about patient's illness, rules of taking medication, alternate treatment options should be discussed thoroughly. This is the right of patient.

In our society, most of the time the daughter-in-law is sent to her mother's house as soon as she is diagnosed as pregnant! People try to establish the concept that the look after of the pregnant lady will be better there.

Both husband and wife are liable to the responsibility of looking after the upcoming child. From the first day if the husband and wife cannot work as a team, it will be difficult for the wife in the long run to get appropriate support from the male partner. Women should be aware of it. Pregnancy is a new experience for women as well as men. Think of it as a team work to be successful.

Few days ago, to get technical assistance of my health awareness programs, I met one high ranked government official and discussed some ideas to improve women's over all health. She did not understand the depth of its need and answered with a satisfactory smile, "We're already working on maternal health." We must remember that "Woman is not only a baby making machine." From policy making to its implementation female health is confused with maternal health. Woman with suboptimum pre pregnant health status cannot be able to conceive/ deliver/ take care a healthy baby.

We see many patients who have offices from 9 to 5. After office due to traffic jam, other house hold responsibilities they could not come to consult doctor at a regular and timely manner. As a result, the disease continue to progress. On the day when she cannot get out of bed due to illness, could not go to the office, that day she came to the doctor. If she came early it could be easy, less costly. For this reason, every workplace should have minimum health checkup facility. It will be better for women if they may have the opportunity of flexible working hour.

Women who are enlightened at present with their glorious contribution to the society crosses over obstacles and go ahead. Mutual communication and cooperation among them should be established. All these efforts can build a society in which men and women will enjoy equal rights and dignity.

Contact:

Website: www.drpurabi.net
E-mail: dr.purabi@yahoo.com
YouTube channel: NowsheenPurabi
Facebook: Dr. Purabi's help desk
LinkedIn: Dr. NowsheenPurabi

About The Author

Dr. Nowsheen Sharmin Purabi is a Gynecologist, writer, teacher, researcher and devoted health awareness activist. She has been serving laboriously for more than one decade to provide door step health services for the women and to build up health awareness among them. Most probably she is the first physician of the country who could be able to send the required messages of health awareness to the interior localities of the country in combined utilization of the mass media, social media and information technology.

She is the planner and presenter of the popular women's health awareness TV shows 'Tonumon' [Mind and Body] in National Broadcasting Media 'Bangladesh Television'. She provides free medical advices in popular social media sites Facebook and Youtube in the name of 'Dr. Purabi's Help Desk'. Focused area of her works are reproductive health, adolescent health, respectful maternity care, safe motherhood, family planning, prevention and control of noncommunicable diseases, nutrition, mental health and first aid.The field level health workers and medical students are also benifitted by her writing, articles and lectures on health issues attached in the webportal.

She is the Brand Ambassador of Microsoft, the world famous technology affairs company, member of International Exchange Alumni (Government Organization of US) and one of the 'Top 10 Health Awareness Activist' listed by 'Linkedin', the largest professional networking site of the world.

She has been working to establish women empowerment side by side with ensuring good health for all.

She is married and mother of a daughter.